VITAL SIGNS

HEALTH IN BORNEO'S SARAWAK

A. Baer, Ph.D.

Borneo Research Council

Occasional Paper Number Three

Borneo Research Council, Inc.

2006

Borneo Research Council Occasional Papers

Published by

Borneo Research Council, Inc.
P. O. Box A
Phillips, ME 04966
U.S.A.

G. N. Appell, Ph.D.
Vinson H. Sutlive, Jr., Ph.D.

Library of Congress Catalog Card No. 2006927847

ISBN 1-929900-08-2

International Board of Editors for Borneo Research Council Publications

Publications of The Borneo Research Council

Monograph Series

Female and Male in Borneo: Contributions and Challenges to Gender Studies. Vinson H. Sutlive, Jr. Editor. 1991. ISBN 0-9629568-0-5.

The Seen and the Unseen: Shamanism, Mediumship and Possession in Borneo. Robert L. Winzeler, Editor. 1993. ISBN 0-9629568-1-3.

Traditional Medicine Among the Ngaju Dayak of Central Kalimantan: The 1935 Writings of a Former Ngaju Dayak Priest. A. H. Klokke, Editor and Translator. 1998. ISBN 0-9629568-7-2.

A Study of Brunei Dusun Religion: Ethnic Priesthood on a Frontier of Islam. Eva Maria Kershaw. 2000. ISBN 0-929900-01-5.

"Never Stand Alone": A Study of Borneo Sociality. Christine Helliwell. 2001. ISBN 1-929900-02-3.

I. H. N. Evans Bornean Diaries 1938-1942. A. V. M. Horton, Editor. 2002. ISBN 1-929900-03-1.

Journeys of the Soul: Anthropological Studies of Death, Burial, and Reburial Practices in Borneo. William D. Wilder, Editor. 2003. ISBN 1-929900-04-X.

Fishing and Headhunting in the Former Culture of Ngaju Dayak in Central Kalimantan. A. H. Klokke, Editor and Translator. 2004. ISBN 1-929900-05-8.

Madness, Death and Ritual in Melanau Ontology. Ann L. Appleton. 2006. ISBN 1-929900-06-6.

Occasional Papers

Social and Behavioral Aspects of Malaria Control: A Study Among the Murut of Sabah, Malaysia. Foong Kin. 2000. ISBN 1-929900-00-7.

Genes, People and Borneo History: A Review. A. Baer. 2005. ISBN 1-929900-07-4.

Please visit the Borneo Research Council Website:
www.borneoresearchcouncil.org

VITAL SIGNS: HEALTH IN BORNEO'S SARAWAK

BORNEO RESEARCH COUNCIL

OCCASIONAL PAPER NUMBER THREE

A. Baer, Ph.D.

Table of Contents

Photographs

ACKNOWLEDGMENTS

This book could not have been written without the help of the dedicated workers in the Sarawak Health Department or without the permission to do fieldwork granted by the Sarawak Planning Unit of the state government. I owe a special debt to Andrew Kiyu, the general facilitator of this work, and to Jayl Langub who provided timely advice on many occasions. A Fulbright fellowship in 2001 also helped.

I thank Mary Huang, Michael Leigh, Patricia Nayoi, Susan Pernia, Clifford Sather, Hew Cheng Sim, Otto Steinmayer, and an anonymous reviewer (on Bidayuh material) for their aid in the project and their input, including comments on sections of the text. I am grateful to the many people who have communicated unpublished information to me; they are acknowledged in the notes to the text. Finally, the friendliness of all the Sarawak people I met made my work both enjoyable and meaningful.

FORWARD

WHO IS WRITING THIS STORY?

This book is about human health in the East Malaysia state of Sarawak, located in Borneo. I have looked at the life of people in towns and villages on the one hand and, on the other, looked at the delivery of health services to them. I have looked at a complex "inside" world.

Since I am an outsider—both an academic and an American—what I have seen, noted, and written is just one interpretation. Because I am a biologist, my account may seem rather broad to some readers. My experience is based much more on the natural sciences and anthropology than on medicine or sociology. Since I can't escape my own background, I had better explain how I happened to take up this challenging project.

Long before I started this study of health in Sarawak, I had studied the indigenous groups called Orang Asli in West Malaysia. This had led me from a human-genetics mindset to a scrutiny of human ecology and culture, from theory-driven research to practical considerations. That early work was largely on malaria. Malaria, as most people know, is a serious problem that involves mosquitoes, parasites, ecology, and human nature—meaning both human genes and human behavior in a humanized landscape. In fact, malaria has been described as being more of a social problem than a clinical disease. In a related sense, the medical arts are now recognized as only one aspect, albeit a vital one, of human health. As such, my hope is that this book will help to harmonize the perceptual worlds of clinicians, scientists of various stripes, and Sarawak communities. Such understanding can foster mutual communication and mutual benefits.

As I came to realize, the complex interaction of people and other living things is basic to the malarial situation, not only in West Malaysia but also in Sarawak. That is, malaria "introduced" me to Sarawak. Colleagues in Malaysia and elsewhere also contributed to my growing involvement with health questions about Sarawakians.

But to talk about "involvement" is quite misleading, given the years I have studied the health problems of Orang Asli compared with the time I have had to study those of Sarawakians. I started looking at Orang Asli health problems in 1971 and Sarawakian ones only in 1995. It was not until 1999 that I began some fieldwork in Sarawak. Even worse, although I had long ago learned to speak one of the Orang Asli languages, I can't claim that asset for any of the indigenous languages of Sarawak. Fortunately, my home language, English, is widely spoken in Sarawak, which has been a boon. In addition, as I will never see 60 again, I hardly expect to be able to spend the next 30 years learning all that I want to know about Sarawak. For one thing, I am no longer skinny and nimble enough to climb muddy mountains or traverse a fallen log spanning a stream. For another, there are so many cultural systems in Sarawak that no one can fathom them all. This book, then, is not definitive.

One thing became obvious to me at an early stage of this project: Sarawak is different from West Malaysia. While both have mountains and mosques, Sarawak still has a few orangutans and West Malaysia a few tigers. However, the orangutans and tigers live on different land masses separated by the wide South China Sea. There is a rumor that if West Malaysian officials had designed Sarawak, they would have put it at the foot of the Malaysian Peninsula, just north of Singapore, so it could be more conveniently controlled by Kuala Lumpur. Stranger than this, Sarawak is almost as large as all of West Malaysia combined, although its population is only 10% that of the Peninsula. It is also true that, on the whole, the indigenous peoples of the two areas are culturally distinct, besides being separated by the sea.

Political history also enters into this picture. British colonialism differed in Malaya and northern Borneo. Malaya made money for London from tin and rubber but Borneo consumed money both in British naval protection and by private-fortune input (before oil was discovered in 1903).[1] The British abetted colonial interests in northern Borneo partly to keep other European powers out.

Beyond that, part of the history behind this account is that I arrived in Sarawak with a Peninsular orientation. (If it had been the other way around, both my Sarawak work and my Orang Asli work would have been notably different.) In coming from West Malaysia, I did not expect that the rural health situation in the two places would be so distinct. For example, Bidayuh and Iban doctors and nurses are not a novelty in the Sarawak Health Department. Among Orang Asli, however, I know of only one who is a doctor, and he is in private practice. All that being said, the two areas do have some similarities in their health situations. For one thing, people in the two areas tend to eat the same kinds of foods and live in similar landscapes. For another, in neither area does rural health receive what could be considered liberal governmental funding, despite the evident economic strength of the country as a whole. Then too, goiter is still a problem in both areas, despite

[1] The first English rajah of Sarawak claimed he spent 30,000 pounds sterling in personal funds on the state (Walker 2002).

the ease and economy of eradicating it. These and other particulars, such as nutritional problems, are discussed in the text.

As is often the case in writings of this sort, I have generally followed a chronological format. This approach highlights what was known and not known in the past and what remains unknown—or at least unpublished—today. It also leads easily to a consideration of current issues and future prospects. One problem with all the sober reports on health and disease is that few outside of the medical profession read them. In the hope that a less formal account would be more palatable, I decided to try that format. If it fails to improve health, it will have a lot of company.

However, no format yet devised can survey topics on which information is inadequate. Getting to the bottom of things in such cases is impossible. In the present context, such orphaned topics include, among others, some sexually transmitted diseases and the health situation of some Orang Ulu (upland) groups. There is always the danger in such cases that "educated guesses" will obscure rather than clarify reality because of the all too human tendency to generalize from insufficient evidence. And yet, limited information can often be counterweighted by looking widely for insights from different social sectors. By combining these different ways of knowing and learning into the text, I have tried to open the door to a broadening of our understanding about health problems.

Despite such defects, I would maintain that conclusions can be reached about the health and disease situations in Sarawak. Such conclusions emerge because the efforts of various workers have produced reinforcing results or observations. The information leading to these conclusions is the core material of this account. While the conclusions I have drawn should be treated cautiously, they tell an important story. That story is fundamental to understanding and applauding the vitality of Sarawak. It might also suggest new opportunities to sustain and improve health in Sarawak and elsewhere.

A Glimpse of Malaysia, Borneo, and Sarawak
for People Who have Never Been There

Kuala Lumpur, the capitol of Malaysia, is rife with philistines, but so is Detroit or Dallas. "KL" has a nifty double skyscraper and a decrepit bus station. The skyscrapers in Detroit and Dallas are shorter, but I don't know about their bus stations.

Malaysian culture is largely rural and forest based. The rural Orang Asli in West Malaysia are the most humane and polite people, thoroughly gentle and

and civilized, which may be the reason that they have become downtrodden.[2] Many groups in Sarawak are like this also. They are wonderfully cheerful in spite of everything.

Malaysian Moslems take pilgrimages to Mecca. Non-Malaysian eco-tourists take pilgrimages to the rainforest. There is a lot of ritual and expense involved in both enterprises. There are also some health risks.

Over the centuries, Borneo has been on the periphery of several empires: Indian, Chinese, and European. The Dutch and British got entrenched in Borneo for a while. Sarawak in northern Borneo was once the fiefdom of a British self-proclaimed ruler, or Rajah. The Second World War led to the downfall of that bizarre experiment. But the Rajah's capitol city, Kuching, is still the capitol of Sarawak. Kuching is an unspectacular city, not yet a vertical one. It is sprawling and livable and sits next to a lazy river. Most of the people in Kuching are practical but some are political.

Whenever I leave the United States for Sarawak, I tell friends I'm going to Borneo. If I say Sarawak, they may think it is somewhere in Eastern Europe. Such innocence works both ways. Not so long ago, when I happened to be in KL, I was asked when I was going back home to London.

According to national statistics, the pluralistic makeup of Sarawak in 2000 was:[3]

Citizens:	
Malays	462,270
Iban	603,735
Bidayuh	166,756
Melanau	117,690
Chinese	537,230
Others	8,103
Non-citizens:	62,738
TOTAL	2,071,506

What does health mean to Sarawakians? To their health workers? Interestingly, there is no word for health in the Bidayuh language or in some others in Borneo. Health/disease is not seen as a dichotomy or as a continuum with two poles. It is multi-dimensional. One's being, or essence, depends on human companionship, a sense of place, traditional rules (*adat*), in addition to healers and individual coping strategies.

What health means to the World Health Organization (WHO) or to Malaysian Ministry of Health may be something else, such as charts showing increased numbers of childhood vaccinations over the years. WHO and Sarawak citizens often seem far apart.

[2] I once asked an Englishman what he meant by "civilized" and got a curious answer, "Tea at four o'clock."

[3] Yearbook 2003.

CHAPTER ONE

THE BEGINNING

Owk, Owk

In an Iban longhouse a three-year old tot smiled at me with decayed baby teeth. One old woman had a conspicuous goiter and an old man had long been blind. These hints of ill health among rural Iban were to me like the first rumble of timber trucks in the Borneo hills—an indication of problems ahead. For like the prelude to serious logging, at first glance the health of rural people seems not to be a large problem. In the towns, on the rivers, in the villages, most Sarawakians look healthy.

On further acquaintance, however, ill health becomes more suspect. One woman tells me of a large lump on her breast. A young Iban father has an infected finger with a blood-suffused fingernail. A nurse has a swollen ankle that she does not know how to cure. A farmer becomes drunk in town, vomits, and—being unable to walk—is shouldered by two women to the local bus to go home. Such things are noticeable. But people's health today is far better than it was a generation ago, according to many reports.

I had first come to Sarawak in northern Borneo in 1968 when the state capitol, Kuching, was only a river town. Few roads existed in the island and most traffic was by water. We took a Chinese coastal steamer, graced by a young cross-dressed passenger, overnight to Sibu and then took a thundering riverboat up the Rejang to Kapit to visit longhouse people. It was the time of the annual Gawai cultural festival, and many Iban were in town, the men reveling in the cockfight competitions. Somehow we drank too much *tuak* and did some off-key singing in a longhouse below the rapids. Sarawak's health problems were far from my mind.

In the 1990s I was back again in Kuching, now a bustling city, because of my general interest in health issues throughout rural Malaysia. I was there only long enough to compile an historical sketch on Iban health gleaned from the city's libraries.[1] Later, in the United States, I gathered more library and internet information on health in Sarawak, and I harvested this bonanza before I returned to Sarawak for a planned field study on health there in several ethnic groups. There were two main drawbacks to this plan: I was unfamiliar with Sarawak's many cultures and I was not a physician. Being a human biologist, I would need to look at health as a component of life in general. This work turned out to be interesting but fuzzy. After seeing a Kuching newspaper that admonished its readers not to be "fuzzy" in choosing a career, I had to admit to myself that trying to be a medical-anthropological ecologist in Sarawak certainly had fuzzy aspects.

Following some studies I had done in West Malaysia on indigenous health problems, I had been invited to do a health review of indigenous groups in Sarawak—in East Malaysia. The idea was that I might manage this in three or four years, rather than the three decades I had taken to study the West Malaysian health problems of Orang Asli ('original people'). So with the guidance of the public health staff of the Sarawak Health Department, as well as the encouragement of cultural experts, I started on this amorphous venture. It was clear to everyone, however, that I would never comprehend all the health variables in Sarawak. I could only hope to "cover the basics".

My first day of fieldwork was somewhat disconcerting. I couldn't understand the local language and, in particular, was mystified by the frequent comment that sounded like "Owk, owk," only learning much later that it meant 'Yes, yes.' Sarawak was not West Malaysia, I reminded myself. Not only were many Sarawak people Christians but, fortunately for me, many people spoke English. And the health workers I met that day were noticeably conscientious.

The first field area I happened to be in was largely populated by the indigenous Bidayuh people, and childhood under-nutrition had long been a problem there. I knew that this Upper Serian area around Tebakang was a place that Alfred Wallace, a household name to biologists and Sarawak historians, saw in the 1850s. He wrote that he had gone up the Simunjan River, a tributary of the Sadong, to "Tabokan" (Tebakang?), which then had a Bidayuh round house for accommodating visitors. Wallace continued upstream to "Borotoi" and "Budw" and then traversed to the head of the Sarawak River via Menjerru (or Menyille, or Menyerig), a village of several Bidayuh longhouses, about 600 feet above a valley. He visited Sodos and Senna (still Bidayuh) then went down the Sarawak River to Kuching.[2]

The Upper Serian area was hilly limestone when I saw it, with "skeletal" soils poor for farming. And the Bidayuh villages I saw were

[1] Baer 2001b.
[2] Wallace 1962.

bunched-up mini-towns, unlike the scattering of hamlets that make up many traditional Orang Asli or Malay villages. Moreover, as it was midday when we arrived at our first village stop, it seemed deserted. Only the numerous dogs napping in the skimpy shade lent an air of familiarity to the scene. Something would have to be done.

The dogs paid no attention to a Euro-American woman, myself, strolling into their territory with an entourage of three medical people. Only when I pulled out my stash of drawing tablets and packages of colored pens on the longhouse verandah did children and a few adults materialize. Luckily, it was a school holiday, so by giving out paper and pens to the milling children I managed to observe them closely. They all plunked down on the bamboo-slat flooring to draw whatever their imagination required, almost as if it were a UNESCO art contest.

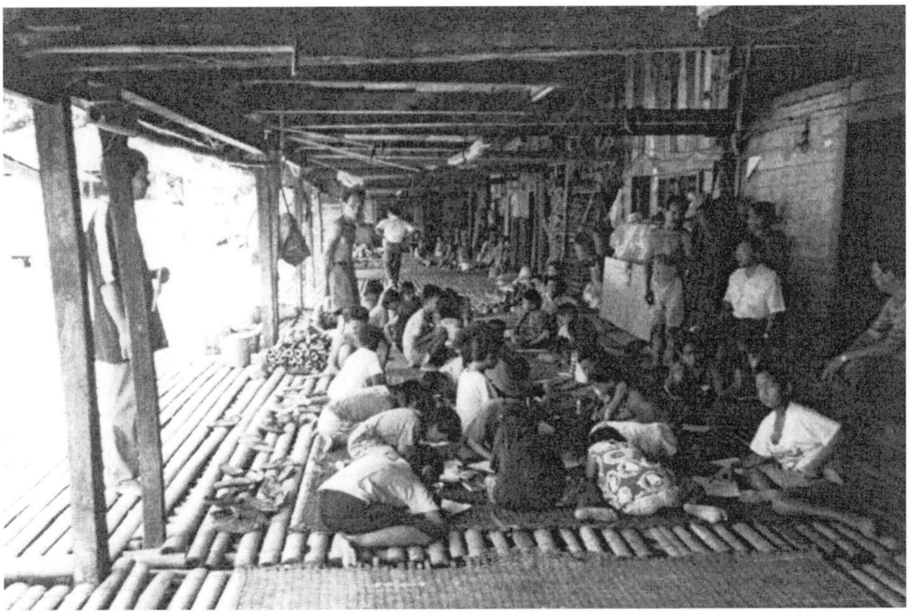

Photograph 1. Bidayuh children drawing pictures at the Tepoi longhouse, Serian District, 1999. The man standing on the left is the village *wakil*, a volunteer health promoter.

While they were preoccupied, I took note of a few pot bellies (intestinal worms? poor nutrition?), one fat boy but many more skinny ones, plus skinny girls. Very few skin ailments, such as ringworm. Black hair, not brownish as can occur with protein deficiencies. Babes in mothers' arms, a bit shy, but plumper than the older children. Several old women, frail and topless, with sunken cheeks and no teeth. There was too much to observe and too many questions to ask.

After a few weeks among the Bidayuh, their health clinics, and their town produce markets, I still had more questions than answers. This was no fault of anyone. It was simply that the reasons for the existing childhood skinniness and stunting were not well understood. And even less was known about old peoples' health. But I persevered, at least in terms of making some guesses (see the later chapter on nutrition). Soon thereafter I had to leave Sarawak, planning to return the next year (2000) and further my questioning—this time on Iban, another indigenous group important to my survey of the state.

I recalled what Alfred Wallace had written in the nineteenth century, that Sarawak's "social and physical conditions are not liable to rapid change."[3] Now, however, rapid social and ecological changes are the norm. One example is that health in Sarawak had been steadily improving for decades, thanks in large part to steadily improving health-care services. Comparing 1970 and 1998, for example, here is the basic information. In 1970 the rate of neonatal deaths, infant deaths, and maternal deaths (per 1,000 live births) were 13.6, 31.1, and 0.9, respectively. In 1998 they were 3.6, 6.2, and 0.2—all showing major declines.[4]

Not Your Typical Tourist

Upon returning to Sarawak in 2000, I knew that I would only have time to see a few Iban. The Iban are a much larger group than are the Bidayuh. At least I had done my homework. I was fortified with "full strength" Iban literature and verbal clues from Iban scholars about the Iban health situation.

I had decided in 1999 that Bidayuh culture, including health, was in a state of flux—untraditional in some ways, unmodern in others. It was, in fact, a work in progress, much like my own Sarawak health survey. Would Iban be the same?

In July of 2000 I spent several weeks among Iban and their assorted neighbors and health workers, in what is now called Sri Aman Division. I saw different Iban lifeways—upriver, downriver, in town, and even at a resort. By good luck, I had brought four pounds of toothbrushes as a gift to an upriver longhouse. Maybe the tot I saw there with decayed baby teeth would get to use one of them, I thought, after learning that no dental team had ever visited there.

At the resort, an Iban waitress flashed me a welcoming smile. To my dismay, I saw that she had brown halos of decay on her top two incisors. I

---

3 Wallace 1962:ix.

4 Tan Chin Siang 2001.

was getting a teeth-problem fixation! Then I remembered Jalil, the young Temuan Orang Asli man who had visited my family in the U.S. years earlier. He noticed that Americans do not have holes in their teeth, unlike people in his village. After going to the dentist and getting his teeth repaired, he said that when he got home he was going to tell his friends that in America adults have perfect teeth. Why? Because when the teeth get decayed, the people there just pull them out and new ones grow again! But since Temuan do a lot of teasing, I knew that no one in his village would believe him.

I decided on the basis of all this to talk about teeth at the divisional health headquarters at the first opportunity. At the same time, I continued to be concerned about poor nutrition in Sarawak—not only its causes but its possible means for improvement.

In the U.S. I had read a book on RAP, rapid assessment procedures. I was impressed by the story of a United Nations worker in Nepal who needed to study potato farming there. He had simply gone to a town market and bought every kind of potato sold. When he emptied his potato sack in his village of study, everyone gathered around and, without prompting, told him all he needed to know: which variety grew fastest, which was tastiest, which was disease-prone, and which produced the largest potato crop.

With this in mind, I had already purchased seed packets of nutritious vegetables that had identifying pictures on them in Kuching, plus some packets of marigolds. The vegetable packets included eggplant, cucumber, three kinds of green beans, and four kinds of spinach and related leafy greens. I would show a "test" array of one packet of each kind in some Iban longhouse and ask which grew best, which was tastiest, and so forth. Then I would tell people they could have a packet each to keep. If many chose marigolds, I would conclude that there was little interest in a balanced diet (or no time available to do gardening). If they preferred beans or spinach, I would probably conclude otherwise.

In the event, the "test" both failed and succeeded. The longhouse group disdained the marigolds entirely. ("Can you eat them?" "Well, no.") And they said all the vegetables grew well and were tasty, which I considered a good sign. When they noticed I had more seed packets in my tote bag, it became obvious I would have to given them all that I had.

Among this longhouse group were my longboat-man and the so-called medical assistant (a paramedic) from the nearby rural clinic. Both of them selected a variety of four vegetable packets for their own gardens and asked if they could keep them. The medical assistant was particularly satisfied with this "test." He smiled contentedly, saying that he would start a clinic garden and it would be a help in combating malnutrition in his remote area. Fortunately this happened just as the Iban were clearing their hill fields for the year's planting season. So my timing was good, even if the "scientific" approach got overwhelmed by practical considerations. But I too was content with the (unexpected) results.

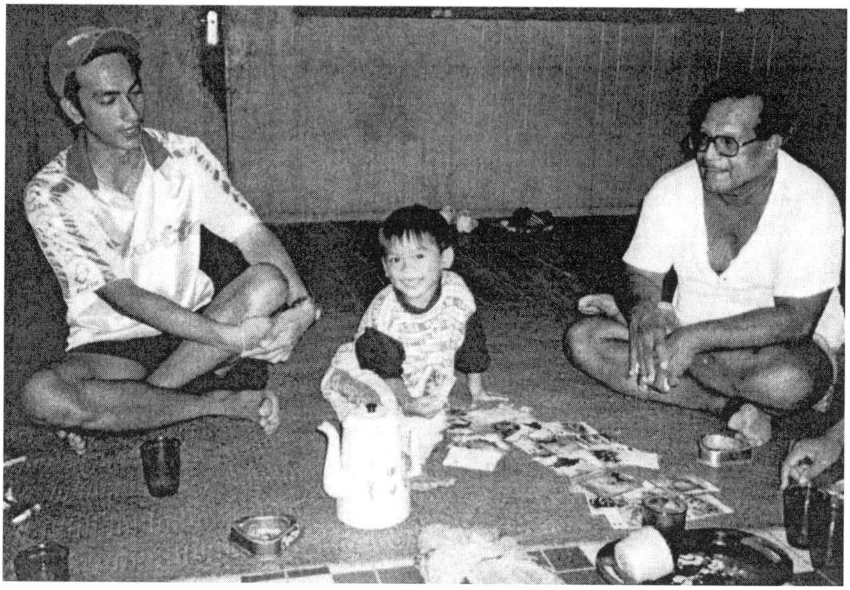

Photograph 2. The "seed packet experiment" at Nanga Delok, with the local medical assistant, Hasbi, on the left of the Iban child and a visiting missionary on the right, 2000.

Parts of my Iban study area in the Sri Aman Division are attractive to eco-tourists. Indeed, I had seen Dutch, French, Australian, Japanese, and American visitors at the local resort. But now I was in Lubok Antu Town, a few kilometers downstream, where outsiders are rarely seen, except for the Indonesians who travel over the mountainous border to sell their produce in this Malaysian market town. Lubok Antuans are largely Iban or Chinese, or both.

The health clinic in Lubok Antu is unusual in that it is in two separate buildings. One houses the medical assistants, all male, who treat general ailments and injuries. The other houses nurses, all female, who are in charge of maternal and child health. The combined clinic serves the town plus 34 Iban longhouses, all being along the road to Sri Aman, the divisional center. Longhouses accessible only by boat are under the purview of other clinics.

Most everyone I saw in Lubok Antu wanted to know where I came from, how many children I had, and, most of all, what I was doing there. These are the usual questions in Malaysia when a pale stranger appears. Once it was established that I was not a missionary but something to do with "medical," I heard about local health problems. A woman had died of malaria because she had waited too long for treatment. A case of suspected Japanese encephalitis had just been found. And many of the oldest town people shuffled along, bent over. (Was this ankylosing spondylitis?) But childhood undernutrition was relatively low in this area, I was told. Only 16%, according to the clinic records for 1999. While 16% was still worrisome, it was much better than the 40% or 50% undernutrition recorded for some Bidayuh areas I'd seen the previous year. Why the difference?

Maybe the brownish soils in this area were better than the acidic, limestone ones Bidayuh farmers in Serian District had to contend with. Or maybe the Iban here had more money from their commercial farming to buy wholesome food? Or were the Iban here better educated? Or none of the above?

One factor did seem to be "easy money." For example, easy-money cars could be seen around the Batang Ai area. They were usually rusted out and abandoned in some ditch. When some upriver Iban were moved downstream to a resettlement area to make way for the Batang Ai dam project over a decade ago, the household heads received a lot of cash to help compensate them for the loss of their traditional land. Not being cash-clever, some Iban squandered it on ephemeral pleasures, including cars that they did not know how to drive well or how to maintain. But these "hydro refugees," according to the health clinic records at Nanga Mepi in the resettlement area, did not have much childhood undernutrition either, only 18% for the year 1999. They did have a lot of hypertension, for unknown reasons. And they drank a lot of cheap liquor in "coffee" shops.[5] For young men, this led to predictable (and preventable) accidents. Gunning their motorcycles after dark to return home along rutted roads, besotted and speeding, they ended up with broken legs or worse, next to a tree that got in their way.

I had been given a friendly warning by someone knowledge-able not to compare the health situation of Orang Asli in West Malaysia with that of Sarawak people. But the temptation was strong on one occasion—all the more so as a tropical storm was raging outside my night's shelter at the time. First, many Orang Asli do not regularly receive the health services that rural Sarawakians do, as far as I know. Second, a large proportion of Orang Asli have been moved off their territorial lands to less salubrious locations, mainly because they are denied land rights. Sarawak, however, is a very large and sparsely populated state and many indigenous people there still live on, and maintain rights to, their customary lands. Moreover, rural Sarawakians are not, in general, as poor as Orang Asli. The paradox

[5] The only health study that surveyed Iban about drinking habits found that 40% of the men drank at least once a week while only 7% of the women did so, with the drinkers being in the younger age brackets (Strickland and Duffield 1999).

to me was that poor nutrition is a chronic problem for both population groups in rural, especially upland, areas.

I had come to think that a key factor in this dual health problem of East and West Malaysia was the current status and workload of women—mothers and grandmothers. Even teenage girls. Although all the Bidayuh, Iban, and Orang Asli were traditionally egalitarian, times were changing fast. And so far, females lagged behind economically, socially, and educationally. But this argument was not interesting to some officials I met, maybe because I was a foreigner who was talking, or maybe because the officials were generally men!

CHAPTER TWO

INFECTIOUS BUGS

The Flying Carpet and Scabies

Richard Halliburton first saw the "wild men of Borneo" in Berlin, in a circus sideshow.[1] He gaped at their dark skin, loincloths, and red-painted faces just like everyone else in the crowd. The two "wild" men in their iron cage even talked.

One ferocious savage said to the other, "Sho' is hot."

The other agreed. "Sho' is."

Halliburton pegged them as Afro-Americans earning a living as impersonators. Later, in his "Flying Carpet"—a biplane, not Sinbad's magic rug—Halliburton did a grand tour of Southeast Asia, even attending a dance party given by Sylvia Brooke in Kuching. He also dropped, via pontoons on his plane, to the landing stage on the Baleh River fronting Temenggong Koh's longhouse. Koh was impressed by the immense bird and asked if it laid eggs. When assured it could lay iron eggs, he wanted it to lay eggs on an enemy longhouse fifty miles upstream. This horrified the local British Resident, who was entrusted with pacifying the "wild" Iban. He diplomatically averted a war by explaining that the exploding eggs would smash the enemies' heads. They would be no good as trophies.

Halliburton, like other instant friends of Sarawak in the 1920s, was no anthropologist, ecologist, or health expert. He did not seem to notice much at Koh's longhouse except that people got drunk during the welcoming dinner, the mosquitoes were lively, and the smoked heads in the rafter stank. But, according to him, in the old days men who had scabies—*kudis buta* in Malay—acted as night watchmen against enemy attacks. Their itchy skin disease tended to keep them awake and alert. A scabies victim could even sell the infection to others who wanted to keep awake during a period of hostilities.

Scabies is caused by a mite that lays eggs which hatch into larvae. They crawl around the skin, causing the itching. Severe scratching can leave

[1] Halliburton 1932.

indelible scars in long-suffering people. Some Southeast Asian people even today, especially children, have the flaky signs of scabies and its telltale scars.[2]

When I was in the Borneo highlands at Bario in 2001, there was a scabies epidemic among the primary school children that quickly spread to the secondary school next door.[3] This was surprising to me because Bario is a forward-looking place with an attentive health-clinic nurse and several notions shops that sell soap as well as snack foods.

Although scabies is endemic in the wet Asian tropics, few adults these days get it. Not only do they bathe often, they use soap if they can afford it. But the residential schools in Bario were an incubator for scabies. Children living in the school hostels had a matron to supervise them, but washing themselves and their clothes and bed things was probably not rigorously enforced. Besides, most Bario adults did not know what scabies was and how it could be cheaply treated with hot water, scrubbing, and soap. Some thought it was an allergy; one mother even contemplated flying her daughter to a doctor in the lowlands for allergy treatment.

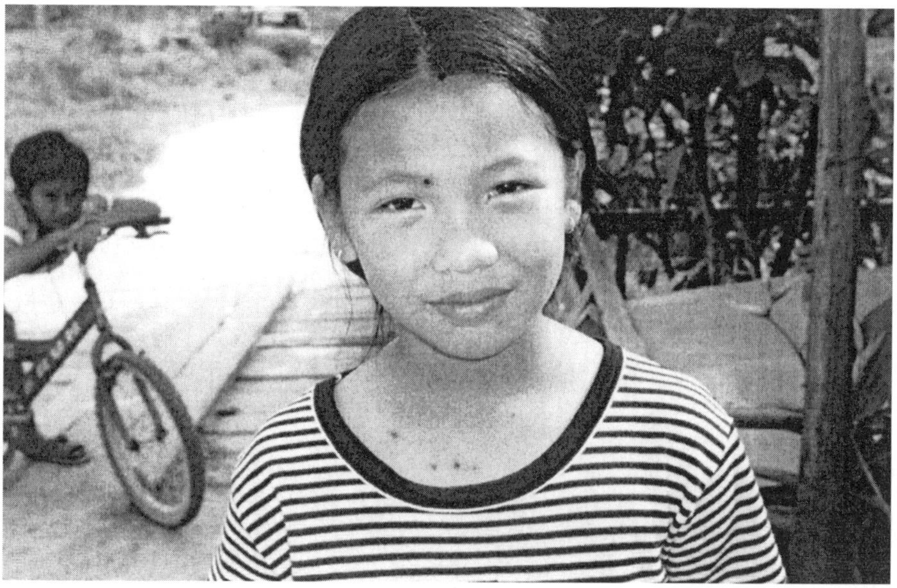

Photograph 3. Gell, a Bario Kelabit girl with scabies, 2001.

[2] In 1984 almost 36,000 new cases of scabies were seen in Sarawak outpatient clinics (Sarawak Medical and Health Services 1986).

[3] Baer 2003.

The school children, rubbing against one another in play and when sleeping, were fair game for scabies. Although the health clinic treated them with a soothing lotion, critical information about combating scabies did not percolate out to the parents, even to those parents close by whose children lived at home rather in the school hostels.

Many hostel children, moreover, left the school on weekends to walk for hours back to their natal longhouse. Those longhouse parents would have little chance to know what the health clinic knew about scabies. Scabies caught at school could then infect distant families, spreading ever outward.

Scabies is a rather benign condition, but it provides one model for thinking about the spread of nastier afflictions in Sarawak today. Scabies is a "flying carpet" that has the hallmarks of information deficits plus human transmission abetted by traditional living conditions that intersect with foreign-modern ideas. Some devastating epidemics also have these hallmarks, spreading insidiously in groups that have no biological or cultural immunity.

Biological immunity is well understood in terms of antibodies and other aspects of the human immune system. It often saves our lives without our even knowing about it. Cultural immunity, in contrast, is caused by behavior or situations that can be fairly localized in a geographical sense. One cultural group, such as the Kelabit or the Lundu Iban, may be largely "immune" to water-borne parasites because they boil their drinking water, while another group may drink water from contaminated sources. Other kinds of cultural practices can confer either immunity or susceptibility for certain diseases.[4]

Mosquitoes, Ecology, and Fevers

It is known that many human ills in the wet tropics were originally non-human forest zoonoses. That is, they were transmitted from one animal host to another, such as by a mosquito. Sarawak is home to at least 86 species of mosquitoes, some of which transmit disease between humans or between animals and humans. Different mosquito vectors of disease can respond in contrary ways to changing land usage. Disease vectors in the environment in the Ulu Suai area of Miri Division were studied from the undisturbed forest phase in 1991 through the development of an oil palm plantation over a four-year period.[5] Anopheles mosquitoes that transmit malaria declined in the area between 1991 and 1994 but the Aedes vectors of dengue virus increased. At the same time, the Culex mosquitoes that transmit Japanese encephalitis virus (JE) did not decrease significantly.

---

[4] Nipah virus borne by fruit bats (an animal reservoir) emerged in Malaysia following land-disturbance modification.

[5] Chang et al. 1997.

The Anopheles species lost out when the oil palm plantation was developed because they breed in shady pool and streams, but the other mosquito species survived in the sunnier environment provided by the plantation. Records obtained from the nearby health center showed that the number of malaria patients declined from 3.6 per thousand population in 1991 to 2.2 in 1994, with 90% of the cases being vivax malaria.[6] (In contrast, vivax made up 67% of the all-Sarawak cases in 1999 and the falciparum type was over 25%, with other categories making up the rest of the reported cases.) While the health center data did not include information on dengue, other available information suggested that the high number of dengue cases recorded in Miri Division in 1993–1994 was caused in part by rural plantations providing habitats for the Aedes mosquito to thrive. In the area under study, these habitats included the water tanks and water-storage jars of the 150 dwelling units erected on the oil palm plantation (no piped water supply having been provided).[7] A lesser concern for plantation areas was JE; while its Culex vector did not decline much in the study area, and while JE viral infection is not rare, few victims develop encephalitis itself.[8] Dengue fevers are more common than JE in Sarawak.[9] An important point here is that since Sarawak has many areas harboring more than one disease-carrying mosquito, any large change in land usage can change the mix of disease vectors and thus the health burden of the local population.[10]

Other factors also affect rates of infectious diseases in commercial plantations, besides the density of disease-transmitting mosquitoes. First, there may be a lack of basic amenities such as piped water supplies, insecticide-treated bednets, and good toilet facilities. Crowding of housing units, immigration of disease-infected workers, and the paucity of domestic animals (which many mosquitoes will bite), are just a few of the variables that can exacerbate these kinds of disease problems. Beyond that, a plantation is an unnatural sight—some would say an unlovely sight.

---

[6] Vivax has long been the major form of malaria in Sarawak; the more severe falciparum malaria is rarer. State-wide, the annual incidence of malaria has usually been below one case per thousand population in recent decades.

[7] Usually, however, this Aedes mosquito (albopictus) breeds in natural pockets of water.

[8] Culex mosquitoes that carry JE prefer outdoor, ground-level victims for biting, especially pigs (Bendell 1970). In 1994 only 26 cases of JE were reported in Sarawak (Chang et al. 1997). Recently a kind of encephalitis similar to JE was found in Malaysia; the causative Nipah virus is a paramyxovirus, while JE (and dengue) are different, both caused by flaviviruses.

[9] In 2003 the Miri blood bank ran low on donated blood because of its use in hemorrhagic dengue fever cases, which were on the rise (Then 2003a).

[10] The mammalian population changes in plantation development have not been well studied. Sylvatic monkeys can be decimated by land clearing; zoophilic mosquitoes that fed on them may turn their attention to new local residents—people. When rats increase in plantations, so do the snakes that eat them. The rats, infected with ectoparasites, can in turn harbor disease threats to people.

What effect this might have on the mental health of the local people is unknown.

A prominent Malaysian was reported as saying that malaria was eradicated in the country long before DDT was banned.[11] In reality, malaria is endemic in Malaysia, with 3,155 cases reported in Sarawak alone for 1999.[12] Most Sarawak cases once were in children, but now adult men predominate. While the number of Sarawak cases seems large, the state-wide incidence is rather low for a Borneo setting. Several hundred of these cases were "imported." When I asked health officials about malaria, I found that they continue to call it a major concern. In part this reflects the immigration of Indonesians from Kalimantan for wage jobs in Sarawak or their visits to Sarawak relatives, especially at festival times. In the Biawak village, on the international border, I was told that both vivax and falciparum malaria occur, the latter coming across from Kalimantan.

Malaria is caused by plasmodial microorganisms that are carried by mosquitoes from the bloodstream of one victim to the next. While bees go to bed at night, mosquitoes do not. Most kinds bite people at dusk or later, although some species prefer to bite animals.[13] The mosquitoes lay their eggs in seepages or puddles or streams, all commonly found in Sarawak.

Iban have long recognized the fever-chill cycle of malaria (*sakit chelap angat*) as dangerous to the body's vitality.[14] In fever, Iban traditionally stayed indoors, under a blanket, to sweat out the heat. In the 1950s high malaria parasite rates were found in the Sarawak interior, with Bidayuh, Kayan, and Kenyah rates being the highest.[15] Malaria rates were correlated with upland areas and with sojourns in field huts during the farming season (with few domestic animals there as alternative mosquito attractants).[16] However, mobile hunter-gatherers had less malaria than did farming groups. As a result of these findings, Sarawak started a malaria control program in 1953 in selected areas. It was later expanded state-wide. When malaria is suspected today, chloroquine is dispensed for three to four days while blood films are analyzed in a clinic or hospital.[17]

---

11 Anonymous 2000b.

12 Anonymous 2000a. In 2001 there were 3,145 cases, with 67% being the vivax kind and 15% being falciparum (Koh et al. 2004).

13 One malaria vector in Sarawak, *Anopheles leucospyrys*, prefers to stay and bite outdoors (Mak 1992).

14 Barrett and Lucas 1993, 1994.

15 De Zulueta 1956.

16 It is still the practice in some areas for whole families to stay in farm huts during the rice season. One example is Nanga Delok, largely a deserted longhouse I found in late July of 2000.

17 Chloroquine is still effective in Sarawak against vivax malaria, the predominant type in the state. However, one medical assistant told me chloroquine plus primaquine is given initially, but if a patient is G6PD-deficient or is pregnant, primaquine is not given. Deficiency in the G6PD enzyme is inherited and primaquine has long been known to cause hemolysis in deficient persons.

Traditional rural dwellings are on stilts, usually on a hill slope with at least one side of the building many feet off the ground. This provides anti-mosquito protection, as they are low flyers and usually bite people in the open at ground level. Hearth smoke also deters mosquito. Fires were, or are, always kept alive in family hearths.[18] The newer ground-level houses fashionable today, with gas cookers, are more mosquito friendly.

Many people sleep under mosquito nets, which in recent times have been impregnated with a mosquito-repelling pyrethroid compound. However, some people sleep in farm huts without these nets and catch malaria there.

For over thirty years DDT was sprayed periodically in houses and in farm huts in Sarawak. The incidence of malaria has therefore fallen markedly in the state, even though areas of ecological disruption remain at high risk today.[19] Also, at the upper reaches of dam-impounded lakes, large areas of stagnant shallows exist among the inlets, conditions favorable for mosquito larvae. This means that longhouses in such locations are mosquito-infested, as I happened to find out in 2000 above the Batang Ai Dam.

Unintended Consequences in Early Vector Control

A Canadian educator in Sarawak in the 1950s under the Colombo Plan wrote, "Shortly before I came to Bario, the World Health Organization undertook a mosquito eradication program to combat malaria in the area, and the spray they used destroyed all the local cats. Before long the place was overrun by rats and the people sent out a distress call to the government. This was before the airstrip was build, and so a helicopter-load of cats in crates was dropped by parachute. Some crates broke open upon landing and the terrified cats disappeared into the jungle in every direction. Fortunately, enough have remained around so that now there is no longer much of a rat problem at Bario."[20]

Vector control via insecticide spraying was the thrust of Sarawak's program against malaria and some other diseases until 1999. But cheaper and often more effective disease-control measures have arisen. Only one, the use of insecticide-treated bednets, has found favor in government circles.[21] Bednets, however, are not a panacea. They will not stop foreigners arriving in Sarawak with new infections. Nor will they stop

---

[18] Melanau burned old, damp sago palm midribs to produce smoke to keep mosquitoes and sand flies away (Hang Tuah Merawin 1994).

[19] For example, the malarial parasite rate in children in the Baram area was 36% in 1952 and down to 3% by 1957 (Colbourne et al. 1989). Other areas showed similar declines.

[20] Toynbee 1997:289.

[21] The history and extent of bednet usage in Sarawak is poorly reported. Bednets have had at least some popularity over the past century, although Geddes (1954) reported that Bidayuh slept under mosquito curtains, not under nets, in 1950.

hunter-foragers from leaving heavy (cotton) bednets behind when they go on forest treks, or stop farmers from doing the same when they camp out in farm huts during the rice-growing season. Moreover, the insecticide permethrin used in treating nets mainly repels mosquitos, forcing them to find victims elsewhere.[22] A related finding from West Malaysia is that treated and untreated bednets are equally anti-malarial over a period of many months, although treated nets are more effective at first.[23]

Some mosquito-borne diseases thrive in urban areas. Sarawak had its first dengue epidemic in 1982 and a year later Lawas District had its own first dengue epidemic.[24] Dengue spread from Lawas Town to villages and schools along the Lawas-Trusan Road, and then to logging camps and upland villages. Most of the victims were children or young adult Dayaks. The severe form of dengue, dengue hemorrhagic fever, occurred in 16% of the cases. The day-biting Aedes vector of dengue was found to be breeding in standing water in discarded junk (bottles, cans), house containers, and in the leaf axils of banana and pineapple plants. Insecticides and an energetic anti-dengue clean-up campaign at the community level helped to end the outbreak. However, this "break-bone" fever continues to afflict Malaysians. In 1996, for example, 14,255 dengue cases were reported, with 32 deaths.[25] In Sarawak, 961 dengue cases were reported in 1998 and 647 in 1999, with about 4% of these cases having hemorrhagic fever.[26] So far, there is no anti-dengue vaccine or drug on the horizon, but most victims of dengue manage to suffer through it.

Southeast Asia has more cases of dengue than any other region of the world, but public awareness is not high. Focus-group discussions in rural Sarawak showed a general ignorance of vector-borne diseases, including dengue.[27]

Filariasis

Filariasis is caused by a nematode, a filamentous worm. Lymphatic filariasis is transmitted by mosquitoes of several sorts and has been fairly common in Sarawak, mainly detected in adults. If left untreated, the adult female worm produces thousands of larvae (microfilariae) daily and lives for many years. This can lead to lymphatic enlargement of a leg (elephantiasis), the scrotum, or perhaps some other part of the body. In Borneo and elsewhere one kind of filarial parasite is specific to humans

[22] World Health Organization 1995; see also Baer 1999a. Permethrin, or the related substance pyrethrin, is also used in Borneo on children to combat head lice. Do treated bednets help counteract lice in Sarawak? They are known to do so elsewhere.

[23] Mak 1994.

[24] Chang and Nagum Jute 1986.

[25] George and Lam 1997.

[26] Anonymous 2000a.

[27] Crabtree et al. 2001.

and is found in many habitats, but the other persists because leaf monkeys (langurs) are "naturally" infected with it and mosquitoes can transmit the disease from them to humans.[28] This latter, sub-periodic kind favors swamp forest. This may mean that filariasis is endemic in Borneo, at least until leaf monkeys become extinct there.

In 1953, 33% of Iban men living in lowland Simanggan (Sri Aman) had filariasis, but few of those living further inland had it. Two of the filariasis victims had scrotal elephantiasis.[29] A survey over 20 years later in Serian District villages found only 5% of the population had microfilariae, but far more males were infected than females in most age groups.[30] People over 50 years of age were most likely to be infected. As no clinical studies accompanied this survey, the elephantiasis rate was not determined. By 1990 filariasis was found in few areas in Sarawak, with only 1% of a surveyed population showing microfilariae.[31] Elephantiasis was limited to just 1.6 persons per 1000 population.[32] However, a newer, more sensitive method of detection recently showed that in endemic districts the prevalence of lymphatic filariasis is about 4%, being equally common in adults and children.[33]

When a friend of mine contracted filariasis in Sarawak I heard about some of the problems in disease treatment. He had experienced inflammation of connective tissue (acute cellulitis), sweating, and dehydration from the *Brugia malayi* type of filariasis. Because this worm has a symbiotic bacterium living in its tissues, antibiotics are needed as a first step to help clear the infection. To kill the worms themselves, a combination of drugs is needed, administered every six months for up to ten years. Until 2003, Malaysia did not import one of the drugs needed to treat filariasis successfully but it started importing it in that year. The aim now in Sarawak is eradication of filariasis in the state. Whether this campaign is successful depends in part on how many native leaf monkeys are left in the state, but immigrants or visitors—whether leaf monkeys or people—could still bring it in.

Typhus

Other bugs besides mosquitoes can carry pathogens that cause fevers. Different forms of typhus exist, scrub typhus transmitted by mites, murine

---

[28] Walsh et al. 1993. Chang et al. 1993, report that other primates plus cats can also transmit filariasis to people.

[29] Griffith 1955. Iban have several words associated with filariasis: *alar*, *dilah rusa'*, *sakit untut*.

[30] Patau Rubis et al. 1981.

[31] Marzhuki et al. 1993. However, in the Upper Tinjar, two longhouses had infection rates of 14% to 16% in 1991 (Chang et al. 1995).

[32] Mak 1992.

[33] Jamail et al. 2005.

typhus by fleas, and tick typhus—by ticks! Sarawak is in the endemic zone for scrub typhus, which can be lethal, but it may be a rare cause of fever in the state, even though its vector occurs in the region. Scrub typhus is rare in Sabah but more common in rural West Malaysia.[34]

Because fevers of unknown origin in Sarawak may be due to typhus, people in the interior of the Rejang watershed were tested for previous typhus infections.[35] They live close to the forest and could have repeated contact with typhus vectors. Blood samples from the Rejang people were laboratory tested to determine if their immune systems had reacted to rickettsia (bacteria) that cause typhus. These tests showed that almost 10% of adolescents and adults had had a typhus infection, including 4% who had been recently infected. Most of the infections were tick typhus, with scrub typhus in second place and murine typhus third. Likewise, among fever patients studied in the Sibu area, two-thirds showed past exposure to rickettsia. Of these, a quarter had been exposed to scrub typhus.[36]

Schistosomiasis

Though rare in Sarawak, schistosomiasis has been found in the Rejang watershed in the area being developed for the Bakun mega-dam. Its vector is a fresh-water snail of swamps and shady forests.[37] The parasite can cycle between the snails and various animals (so-called reservoirs), not necessarily including people. Village dogs may become infected, easily making humans more vulnerable. Fortunately, the disease symptoms in Sarawak have been mild and most people seem to be "dead ends" for the parasites, as they do not excrete schistosome eggs. However, with ecological changes, schistosomiasis might spread and become more severe—as has been the case elsewhere where large dam projects have occurred.

DPT (Diphtheria, Pertussis, Tetanus)

In 1979 a diphtheria epidemic hit Iban children. The disease spread because too few children had had DPT booster shots, but by the mid-1980s 97% of the children studied in the Kapit area were getting their immunizations on schedule.[38] Today DPT immunization is virtually universal in Sarawak.

---

[34] Taylor et al. 1986.
[35] Sagin et al. 2000.
[36] Tay et al. 2000.
[37] Sagin et al. 2001.
[38] Benster and Stanton 1989.

Leprosy and Tuberculosis (TB)

Leprosy is an old story in Sarawak. Recent research shows that one strain of leprosy microbes spread throughout all of Asia many thousands of years ago. Edwin Gomes wrote in 1911 that in one advanced case of leprosy, an Iban woman was exiled to a hut apart from the longhouse; normally people brought her food and water but sometimes she was neglected for days. After the Japanese occupation of Sarawak, new drugs became available to treat and cure leprosy, but the stigma of being a leper remained in the Borneo air. Few cured lepers were welcome in their natal villages.[39] Even in the 1980s, while Bidayuh recognized the symptoms of leprosy, most did not know the cause was a bacterium. Some 23% blamed it on "wrong" foods, weakness, or "dirty" blood, even though it was widely known to be infectious.[40]

Both leprosy and TB, a worldwide killer, can be transmitted directly from person to person, without some vector intervening. Both are bacterial diseases. Sarawak started a leprosy control campaign in 1974. By the mid-1980s perhaps 2,000 or more cases existed in the state; many cases went undetected until people's deformities became obvious.[41] Survey data showed that cultural groups in the interior had three times more leprosy per 100,000 population than did Malays, Melanau, or Bidayuh, while the rate in Iban was about two times that of Malays.[42] Leprosy was more common in situations where people lived in close contact in longhouses, rather than living in detached houses. The same result was found for tuberculosis; crowding fostered TB transmission. Today leprosy is disappearing from Sarawak, thanks to antibiotics and other factors, but TB remains a large concern.

Respiratory problems generally increase with age. For Iban in one study, 30% of the men and 20% of the women under age 40 had respiratory problems but 46% of the men and 34% of the women over 40 had them.[43]

Sarawak's TB control program was started in 1961. It includes BCG (Bacille Calmette-Guerin) vaccination of children, identifying cases, and treating victims. BCG coverage is now virtually 100% in Sarawak children. The incidence of TB cases was 90 per 100,000 population in 1997.[44] A few years later, TB was still worrisome in Sarawak with 40 infectious cases per 100,000 population, even though this was an improvement over earlier years. In one small study, spinal TB was found

---

[39] Calder 1954.
[40] Chen 1988a.
[41] Chen 1988a; Goldblatt 1999.
[42] Chen 1988b.
[43] Strickland and Ulijaszek 1993.
[44] http://sarawak.health.gov.my/

to cluster in older Iban men.[45] Treatment for TB must be continued for months to effect a cure, but some Sarawakians do not "stay the course."

Gastroenteritis and Cholera

While stomachaches are usually mild, diarrheal diseases, often caused by *E. coli* bacteria or a rotavirus, they can present complex problems.[46] In young children they can lead to death, but survivors of an acute phase of undernutrition brought on by the infection can still face growth and development deficits. Poor sanitation fosters diarrhea but effective treatment is widely available in Sarawak these days, such as oral rehydration and antibiotics.[47] However, a recent study in Miri found extensive antibiotic-resistance in *E. coli* isolated from diarrhea patients.[48]

Among 533 Song and Kanowit Iban children up to ten years of age studied in the 1980s, 19% had diarrhea, 27% had respiratory problems, and 5% had fever. The children's total morbidity was 51%. The adults in the study had lower morbidity, 39%, but still a significant amount.[49]

Cholera is an old disease caused by Vibro bacteria that thrive in the in-shore marine environment. It and smallpox were once a "common curse" in Borneo. The symptoms of cholera are acute diarrhea with rapid dehydration, and mortality can be high. Survivors may become asymptomatic carriers of the bacterium, leading to future outbreaks.

Cholera is mainly spread by fecal-contaminated water or by seafood. Surprisingly to me, a recent report details the finding of Vibrio in city markets at all seasons in Malaysia.[50] Cockleshell mollusks were most heavily laden with Vibrio and Kuching had the highest level of seafood contamination of the eleven sites studied. Yet Kuching and other cities in Malaysia do not have cholera epidemics every day. The explanation may involve a complex interaction between the Vibrio normally living in the marine environment, water conditions on land during droughts, methods of cooking seafood, and other factors in human ecology about which I know far too little. However, pathogenic Vibrio can persist for a long time in brackish or ocean water, especially in copepods and other zooplankton, and coastal currents can carry it from port to port.[51] Cholera can thus spread quickly. In fact, the most common strain of Vibrio found in Malaysian city markets, called 0139, originated near Bengal within the

---

45 Rasit et al. 2001. Rates in some Iban areas have been much higher than the national average.

46 A Malaysian child has about a 2% chance of contracting rotavirus diarrhea before reaching five years of age (Hsu et al. 2005).

47 Barker et al. 1988.

48 Wan et al. 2003.

49 Strickland and Ulijaszek 1992.

50 Elhadi et al. 2004.

51 Colwell 1996.

last decade or two and subsequently spread west around Malaysia and up to China. The Malaysian area, with its high rainfall, is "fertile ground" for Vibrio because it favors warm water (shallow seas and estuaries) where zooplankton have abundant phytoplankton to eat and are themselves eaten by fish and other marine animals. El Nino events and gradual global warming are even more favorable for Vibrio's future success in causing disease.

There are reports of cholera epidemics in Sarawak throughout the past 150 years.[52] The epidemics have favored the dry season of May through July, generally in coastal areas where Malay villages are located along the tidal reaches of rivers. Epidemics occur where water supplies, toilet facilities, and personal hygiene are poor. In 1902 cholera caused over 1500 deaths during a drought.[53]

The Cholera Expedition of 1902

To consolidate his one-man rule of Sarawak, in June, 1902 the Englishman Charles Brooke sent his son Vyner Brooke to lead hundreds of Malays and thousands of Iban upriver against autonomous longhouses hostile to his regime. Cholera appeared in the lowlands before the punitive expedition started and it haunted the armada up the river. The many sickened members of the expedition fled home in panic, taking cholera with them and spreading it far and wide. Over 1,000 people died and many more were stricken. The autonomous upland groups escaped the disease because they shunned the dead bodies of the lowlanders.[54]

A cholera epidemic in the 1920s triggered Kelabit dispersal in the highlands.[55] But it still strikes willy-nilly today, even far inland. No cholera cases were reported in 1984 or 1985 but three outbreaks occurred in 1986, one covering six villages in Serian District, another in the same district in Tebedu, near the Kalimantan border, and a third in Kalaka District.[56] Only ten people in all were clinically ill in 1986, a vast improvement over what would have been the case in an outbreak decades

[52] Toynbee 1997; Yadav and Chai Meng Chee 1990. According to Wells (1925), Malays who had bought a bottle of Mecca well water, brought it home to Malaya so that their relatives could drink it and go to heaven; "It is said that...the drinker often gets cholera and probably goes" (p. 166).

[53] In that era, cholera victims were deserted by all and had to fend for themselves—an extreme form of quarantine. Smallpox victims might be cared for by those who had already recovered from it but other people fled to forest shelters. Many victims died when no one would feed them. Smallpox and cholera epidemics killed in the hundreds "on all sides," according to Gomes (1911:201). Generally in such epidemics many deaths occur because too few adults are healthy enough to be good care-givers. That is, the social fabric collapses.

[54] Sutlive and Sutlive 2001.

[55] Bulan 2003.

[56] Sarawak Medical and Health Services 1986.

earlier. Dysentery (amebic or bacterial) can spread as cholera does, by fecal contamination. While it caused much infant mortality in the past, it was not the general scourge that cholera was.[57] Betel-chewing is said to be effective against dysentery in adults.[58]

Like cholera and diarrhea, typhoid is another water-borne disease. In the Limbang District, all three diseases occurred when gravity-fed water pipes were empty during the dry season, the diseases usually hitting the young and the aged.[59]

Some viral hepatitis, a liver infection, has also been associated with poor sanitation, specifically fecal-contaminated drinking water. But hepatitis viruses, a diverse group, can also be spread by contaminated blood supplies and by other means. Hepatitis B virus is said to have over a million carriers in Malaysia, most of them asymptomatic. Neonatal mother-child transmission is suspected. This virus is most prevalent in Sarawak, and especially in Dayak and Chinese communities.

Changing Times

In the past, people were hard put to escape mosquito-borne diseases almost anywhere in Sarawak. Coastal areas were rife with filarial parasites while malaria haunted the interior. Dodging these parasites still left many people at risk of viral or bacterial parasites, let alone intestinal worms. Diarrhea and dysentery were continual problems. Epidemics of smallpox, typhoid, malaria, and cholera once cycled in the Rejang area.[60] Pathogenic bacteria were not far behind, leaving TB and other infections in their wake. Smallpox and measles viruses periodically swept inland from the coast to highlands. Smallpox, in particular, caused social chaos and many deaths. The Brooke dynasty was not conscientious about providing smallpox vaccinations.[61]

Already in the 1930s the League of Nations Health Organization was warning about the effects of modernization on mosquito-transmitted diseases, words that still resonate today:

> Steps must be taken in future to see that the construction…of roads and other engineering works and timber felling shall

---

[57] An epidemic in the 1960s produced twelve deaths, half in small children (McKay and Wade 1970).

[58] Knapen 1998.

[59] Heyser 1992.

[60] Sutlive 1978.

[61] However, when smallpox struck Dalat in 1881, a resident officer noted that the Dalat people had earlier refused to be vaccinated. Only after 1918 were medical dispensaries opened in the Mukah to Dalat area (Morris 1997).

> not create breeding places for the [mosquito] larvae over what are sometimes considerable areas.[62]

Today, smallpox has been eradicated and bacterial diseases respond to antibiotics, at least the newer ones for which the parasites have not yet built up resistance. But animal reservoirs for diseases like measles (non-human primates) and filariasis still exist in nature. Although records show that Sarawak had a major outbreak of measles in 1983 with 2,305 cases reported, increasing measles vaccination has generally kept epidemics of it at bay in recent years.[63]

And new viruses, such as SARS in 2003 or avian flu virus more recently, continue to crop up.[64] (The last flu pandemic occurred in 1968, less than 40 years ago.) Vigilance against these and other disease organisms is the byword. Luckily, Sarawak has no rabies, plague, yellow fever, or polio, as far as I know.

---

[62] Anonymous 1937:78.

[63] Sarawak Medical and Health Services 1986.

[64] SARS is severe acute respiratory syndrome.

CHAPTER THREE

NUTRITION: INPUT, OUTPUT

Malaysia emphasizes exoticism for its first-world tourists and mass culture for its own people. When the tourists come to look at Sarawak they are shown a bustling city, a rain forest, proboscis monkeys, and an awesome cave. When government people look at Sarawak, I think they see "progress." If they travel to remote areas without city amenities, they bring city ideas with them. They approve of ornamental plants around rural houses and rows of whitewashed stones by health-clinic parking lots.

> White Rocks
>
> What do whitewashed rocks signify? Maybe cleanliness, maybe civilization as opposed to nature. Nature is transformed into neatness, wildness is tamed. A Chinese or Japanese gardener would have other ideas, seeing natural rocks scattered around as pleasing parts of a landscape. And in the past, natural rocks were used in Borneo for important cultural purposes, as in the impressive megaliths of Kelabit country.[1]
>
> Whitened rocks today in rural Sarawak, sometimes with used tires positioned neatly near by, may be the aesthetic vision of urban visitors, as may bare-earth vistas around rural dwellings. While a rainforest lacks human control, a tidy longhouse may signify not only victory over nature but transformation of "natural" people into citizens. Planting oil palms in rows on raw earth serves the same transforming end—regimentation. There are no straight lines for plants in nature, and no bare earth in a rainforest, normally. Logging tracks do produce bare earth, sterile and rutted, with down-slope sheet erosion where the hillside has been leveled for the roadbed. After strong rains, landslides create more bareness and inevitably more run-off and river siltation. Do people with an ideology that nature is bad even prefer brown rivers to clear-flowing ones?

[1] The megaliths, also found among related groups in Sabah and East Kalimantan, were part of burial rites (Bulan 2003).

Even if one looks beyond this landscaping, malnutrition and other health problems can be hard to see.

The Ecology of Nutrition

Questions about health, wherever they start, lead back inevitably to nutrition. The starting point may be economics, agriculture, the birth rate, alcoholism, or epidemiology. In every case, if nutrition is not a central concern, many other endeavors fail. It's not that "we are what we eat," but that we are all prone to problems if food is not wholesome and sufficient. The most vulnerable are underfed infants and children because a poor diet cheats the growing body and brain of fulfillment into adulthood.

Sarawak populations are expanding at the same time that food-farming, hunting, forest foraging, and fishing are in decline. A mixture of these activities once provided a balanced, if lean, diet because a diversity of ecosystems provides adaptive resilience unattainable in a blanket of oil palm schemes.[2] In reality, every longhouse was an ecological unit. Now with short fallowing, erosion, river pollution, export-driven agriculture, and forest destruction, farmers can experience not only poor food harvests but also nutrient-poor diets. New food habits, such as eating store-bought snacks, are also noticeable.[3] With these trends, nutritional security may be lost for families, unless wage labor fills the gap.[4] If this scenario applies to many Sarawak people today, nutrition becomes a vital factor both in economic terms and in terms of health care.

Another factor in the nutrition equation, with wage work fairly common, is that little time is left for gardening, fishing, foraging, or basic farming. And with some farmers emphasizing perennial cash crops, land for growing food shrinks. Moreover, oil palm and pepper, let alone rubber, are hardly food staples. With this trend to cash cropping, farmers end up buying more of their food.[5] Who, then, will grow this food?

Only a minority of Sarawak villages today live in a traditional environment. Those that do enjoy a varied diet free of pesticides. For example, botanical work at Nanga Sumpa above the Batang Ai reservoir showed that 160 plant species were eaten there, many of them forest plants. This longhouse also used 105 varieties of rice, 8 of maize, 16 of

---

[2] For Kelabit at Pa Dalih in the 1990s most of their high-protein foods came from wild species, primarily mammals (over 15 species) and fish (15 species). In addition, 33 species of wild vegetables were eaten, plus many kinds of mushrooms (Christensen 2000).

[3] Batang Ai resettlement women interviewed by Hew and Kedit (1987) said they often bought snack foods such as soft drinks and sweets, one aspect of commercial malnutrition.

[4] Even in the early 1990s, 11% of rural families lacked necessities such as food, clothing, and housing (Taylor et al. 1994).

[5] When Bidayuh in the Padawan area said they spent the majority of their cash earnings on food in the 1980s, that meant that they bought canned goods, cooking oil, and rice—not green vegetables or fruits (Burgers et al. 1991).

cassava, and 7 of ginger.[6] In the 1980s the Kenyah of Long Selatong got over 60% of their food from non-domesticates—from the river, from hunting, and from foraged plants; farm crops made up the rest.[7]

A generation ago, few Bidayuh had gardens to provide green vegetables year-round.[8] This is still the case in many Bidayuh and other areas. Few ornamental plants around houses today are edible. There's no place for either kitchen or swidden gardens in an oil-palm plantation or a pepper-vine field. Some Bidayuh villages have their houses packed close together and the people pour concrete all around their living areas.[9] And vegetables don't grow well on a Melanau tidal swamp or an eroded limestone hillside in Serian District.

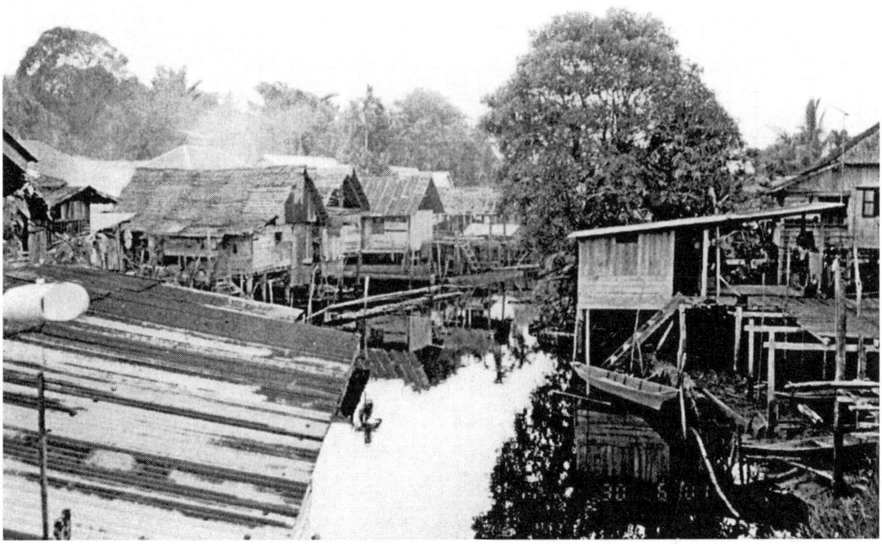

Photograph 4. Kampung Tellian, near Mukah, a Melanau village that was the center of the Brooke-era sago industry, 2001. This coastal swamp is not a good habitat for home gardens.

---

[6] Christensen 1997.
[7] Chen 1985.
[8] Grijpstra 1976.
[9] However, Bidayuh villages like Gayu in Upper Padawan have many well-spaced houses surrounded by vegetable gardens and fruit trees.

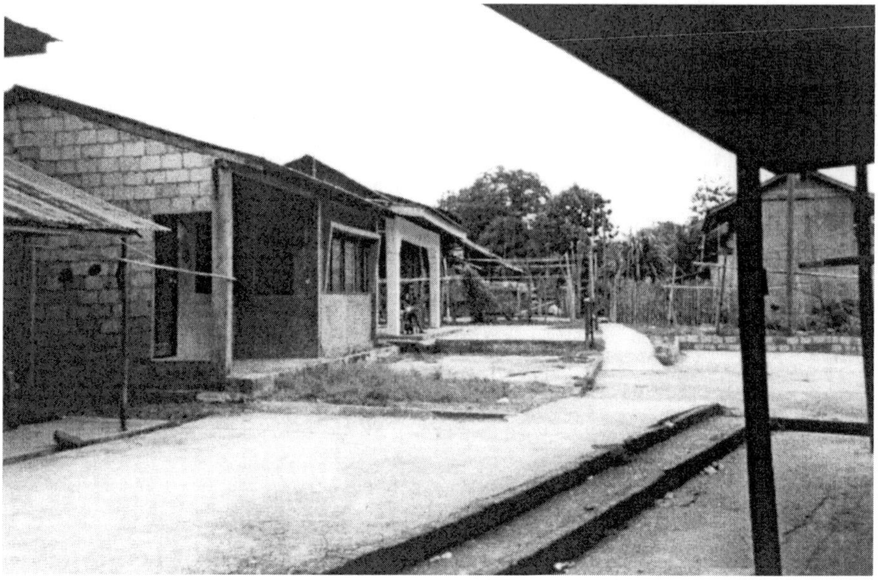

Photograph 5. Temong Bangun, a Bidayuh village in Serian District, modernized with concrete but not having an edible landscape, 1999.

Vegetable gardens are, in theory, encouraged by some government departments.[10] In practice, besides lack of suitable space, social changes are unfavorable for them. In fact, the vegetable and rice growers I've seen were mainly older women. Even then, they *sell* much of what they grow. Many younger people are busy elsewhere, some living far from a self-sustaining, edible landscape. Notably, the preschool at Biawak had an attached vegetable garden when I was there, although school areas that I saw elsewhere had no gardens.[11]

[10] The Agriculture Department tends to focus more on cash crops than on food crops for home consumption. It also talks in terms of fertilizers, pesticides, and weedkillers more than cover plants, intercropping, or agroforestry (Burgers et al. 1991). However, as one man said, "Weeds grow better with fertilizer."

[11] As early as 1977, all six primary schools in the Tebakang area had demonstration gardens. Besides teaching the children the nutritional value of foods, the children could take vegetables home at times. These included okra, kangkong, changkok manis, Chinese radishes, green beans, pumpkins, spinach, cucumbers, eggplant, yams, sweet potatoes, peanuts, and cassava. The schools also grew fruit such as citrus, banana, coconut, rambutan, pineapple, durian, and jade fruit. All schools raised chickens and four of them had fish ponds (Anonymous 1978). According to Talla (1979), the bunds of Bario rice paddies were once planted with vegetables when the rice plants were young. When I was there, however, the bunds were mowed with modern grass trimmers, even though they are built up of fertile muck from the paddies and could support an edible landscape.

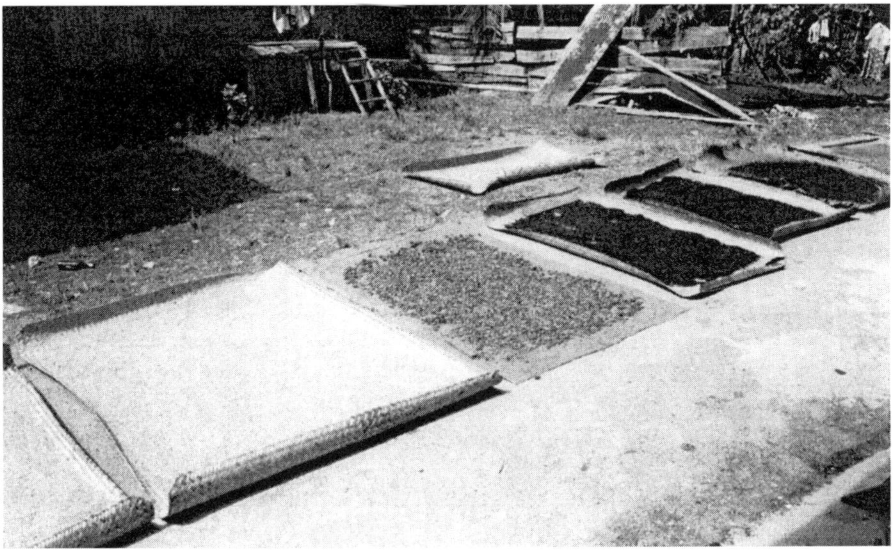

Photograph 6. Rice, cocoa, and pepper drying on mats in Biawak village, Lundu District, 1999.

Above all, when rural men are away on wage jobs and women at home are the full-time crop farmers and caretakers, they have little time for growing vegetables year round. If there is little money to buy them, family nutrition may suffer. Few areas of forest are left for people to forage for fruits, nuts, tubers, sago pith, and so on.[12]

Fruit can substitute for vegetables to some degree.[13] Fruit trees are still found in many village areas, and former longhouse sites often conserve groves of fruit trees. Although fruits such as durian or pineapples may be grown for sale, smaller fruits tend to be for home consumption. The Iban headman at Nanga Delok noted that they needed more fruit trees around their longhouse. But in one Bidayuh village with no fruit trees in sight, a medical assistant said that they discouraged people from having trees within a village. In addition, Lahanan longhouses have been encouraged to remove shading fruit trees, in order to make the compound "look tidier."[14] This pressure ignores the health benefits of both the fruit and the cooling shade provided for living quarters (often with hot, metal roofs these days).

[12] Before the Batang Ai resettlement, over 90% of the women foraged for wild foods at least weekly, but afterward, with no forest nearby, ferns and other wild vegetables were no longer available (Hew and Kedit 1987). The re-settlers found the new area poor for both gathering and growing food (Ayob and Yaakub 1991).

[13] Nutritious fruits, high in protein and potassium, include *dabai*, *kembayau*, *durian nyekak*, and *durian kuning* (Voon Boon Hoe et al. 1999); the first two are olive-like fruits and durian is the famous large, smelly fruit with a pineapple-cream-onion taste.

[14] Alexander and Alexander 1993.

Moreover, the fruit of the small but graceful rambutan tree is a great favorite with children. They scramble up the tree to pick the fruit, which looks something like a red sea urchin with a boiled egg inside but tastes delicious. Much has been lost in the name of tidiness, it seems.

Fishponds have been encouraged in some villages.[15] Later on, those I saw were dry holes, the fish gone—whether dead, eaten or sold. If such a pond were connected to an animal pen and a vegetable garden near by, the integrated system could be more productive and sustainable. In Laos, for example, "The animal manure fertilizes the garden and feeds the fish, and water from the pond irrigates the garden."[16] Fish farming, however, has been a useful innovation in the upper reaches of the reservoir behind the Batang Ai Dam. It provides a much-needed source of protein for the local people.[17]

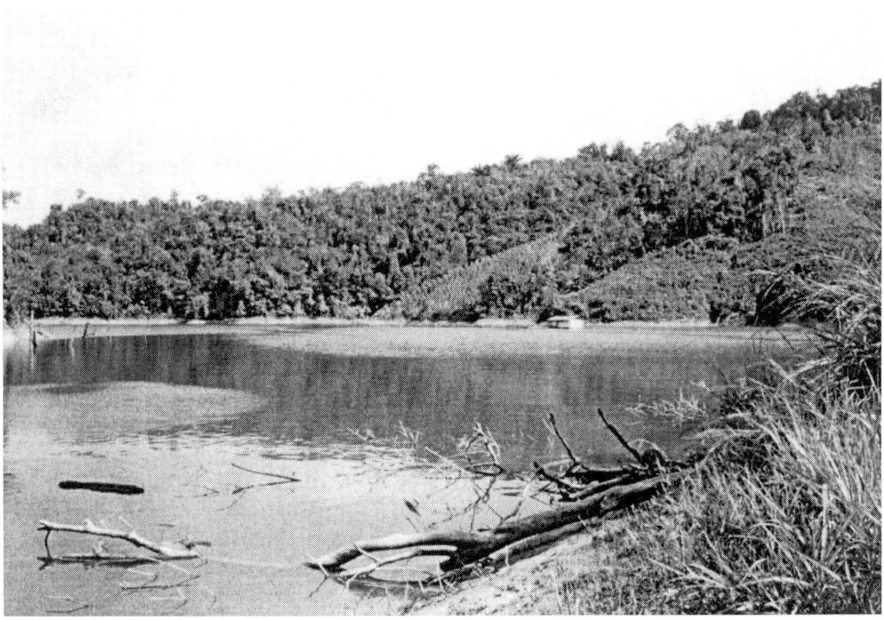

Photograph 7. Fish pen area (white building) in the shallows of the Batang Ai Reservoir. Pepper plot on hillside to the left of the white building, 2000.

[15] Grijpstra (1976) discusses various types of fishponds.

[16] Ireson 1996:249.

[17] According to Horowitz (1998), much of this fish, raised in pens, is sold for cash; this was denied by local Iban in 2000.

Domestic animals kept for home consumption are not abundant throughout Sarawak, at least the parts of the state that I've seen.[18] Even then, they may be sold rather than eaten. Also, a few chickens or ducks around a longhouse could never supply an egg a day for everyone. Water buffalo are scarce except in some highland areas. The buffalo are still used for preparing rice paddies but with traditional feasts now mostly out of fashion, and values changing, they are usually viewed as an investment.

In the nineteenth century Alfred Wallace observed that when cloud galleons race in from the sea, tropical hillsides no longer covered by dense forest are washed away by the rains, leaving great areas of denuded clay and rock. He predicted the extinction of tropical plants and animals if governments and institutions were remiss about saving them. Wild game was plentiful throughout Sarawak in the nineteenth century, when population was sparse and when men (and women) hunted with dogs and spears, or with blowpipes or traps. But no more.[19] (Dogs once helped feed people but now people feed dogs.) Roads, outboard motors, and shotguns have made it possible even for city people, let alone loggers in forest camps, to go hunting afield.[20] A dramatic increase in hunting occurred in Sarawak over the past generation. One logging camp obtained 1,149 animals, or 64,000 pounds of wild meat, in one year.[21] And following logging, even more outsiders penetrate wild areas via access roads. However, by 1990 the loss of wildlife in Sarawak due to logging gave rise to a ban on selling wildlife and wildlife products in the state.[22] In addition, there is now much less natural habitat to sustain deer, wild pigs, monkeys, and other edible animals. A few areas in the uplands still are the haunts of pigs and the like, but deer, for instance, formerly eaten at feasts in the Kelabit area, are no longer plentiful there.[23]

---

[18] One Bidayuh family raised doves, to sell and to eat. But when the government gave chickens to a village elsewhere, they were all eaten in three months, I was told.

[19] Alfred Wallace, among other British Empire explorers in the nineteenth century, found Sarawak irresistible for collecting plants and animals he could sell in London. By selling 5 Sarawak orangutan skins (preserved in arrack) and 16 orangutan skulls he was able to pay his field expenses in Indonesia for a long time (Wallace 1962). In all he killed and caught 17 of these primates and bought 2 more in Sarawak. This occurred near Simunjan in 1855, in a swampy area that today has no orangutans.

[20] One estimate is there are 60,000 shotguns in the state (Horowitz 1998).

[21] Bennett 2000.

[22] Bennett 2000. I do not know if this ban is rigorously enforced, but it needs to be, both for the benefit of local people and for sustaining the priceless diversity of wildlife in Sarawak.

[23] For the devastating effect of logging, cash-sale hunting, and road hunting on wild game, see Dahaban et al. (1996), Bennett (1994, 2000). The protein supply for rural people plummets because they are deprived of wild meat.

Rivers, swamps, and other freshwater sources once contained many edible frogs, turtles, snails, fish, and other animals.[24] Most of these have declined and some contain toxic pollutants these days. Many rivers are "dirty" with sediments.[25] Most aquatic foods now come from the sea in Sarawak but few of them are available far inland except for salt fish, primarily anchovies.

Mega-projects like the Bakun Dam in Belaga District can start a cascade of health problems. While the government provides health services to the many longhouses downstream of the project, the longhouse people have experienced food scarcity, including a decline in fish and wildlife, as well as depletion of potable water and also monsoon flooding resulting from ecosystem changes caused by the dam.[26]

The main staple throughout Southeast Asia is rice, often grown in rain-fed hill fields using only manual labor. Burning off the vegetation on a new field produces ash, the only fertilizer traditionally used. Because the soil is untilled and tree stumps are not removed, erosion and leaching of nutrients are minimized, but yields are often too low for year-round sustenance for expanding populations. Moreover, fuel-driven rice mills these days remove the seed coat, rich in vitamins and minerals.[27] This polished rice is less tasty than traditional mortar-pounded rice that is only half polished. In contrast to hill rice, naturally-irrigated swamp rice requires no field burning or fallow period and gives good yields, unless flooding or drought occurs, but unlike hill fields, does not permit intercropping with vegetables. The irrigation-ditch rice grown in Bario, at 1200 meters in elevation, also gives good yields.

Some Nutritional Data Related to Ecology and Other Factors

The nutritional status of Sarawak people was reviewed in 1999.[28] For children under six years of age, 33% were moderately or severely underweight in 1982 versus 19% in 1995.[29] This huge improvement was unevenly spread

[24] Bintulu Iban, for example, voiced concern about water pollution, declines in wild fish and game, decreases in natural resources for local use, poor health due to dirty drinking water—largely the result of commercial logging (King 1996).

[25] Upriver from Bintulu on the Batang Kemena, the sediment load in September, 1992, was found to be over twenty times the level permitted by the Malaysian Department of the Environment (Taylor et al. 1994).

[26] Then 2003b.

[27] This rice bran, once eaten by free-ranging chickens and pigs when hand milling was the norm, is often a waste product of rice mills. In Bario, burnt husks from rice mills are sometimes spread on fields as a kind of organic fertilizer, I was told.

[28] Duffield and Strickland 1999.

[29] In the 1980s the malnutrition rate was at least twice as high in rural areas as in urban ones. In 1982 it was higher in the pre-school age group (56%) than in toddlers (38%) or infants (14%) (Sarawak Medical and Health Services 1986).

across the state, with some areas lagging far behind.[30] For example, in 1988 Iban children living in a zone of extensive logging were compared to Kayan children living in an un-logged area.[31] While 22% of the Kayan children were undernourished, 78% of the Iban children studied were undernourished. In the same decade, 50% of Iban children under 6 years of age in the Entabai area were underweight and 25% were stunted.[32]

A unique study in the 1990s on an urban squatter community in Kuching showed that 48% of children up to 12 years of age were underweight and another 13% were severely malnourished. More children over 2 years of age were malnourished than were younger children. Iban and Bidayuh children were more often malnourished than Chinese children there.[33] In contrast, children under the age of 5 years in Selangau, which once was an Iban squatter camp near Sibu but is now a town on a main road, had only 16% severe plus moderate malnutrition in 2000.[34]

Few data are available for Sarawak adults. In 1866 Odoardo Beccari was astonished to discover an obese man from the Balui, a Kayan chief named Kam Diam. Even in the 1980s travelers in Borneo were hard put to find fat people, but today the world market of sweets has had a pronounced effect. In Song and Kanowit areas, the proportion of Iban adults who had chronic energy deficiency increased from 16% to 19% from 1990 to 1996 but the proportion of overweight adults also increased, from 13% to 17%.[35] This study showed that the trend toward obesity was pronounced in those living in urban areas and for younger people. Older people, particularly women, were appreciably thinner. By older, I mean over 60 years of age, but "old" is a slippery term; in the 1980s the Iban of Kapit considered Dana, their headman, to be old. He was all of 40 years then.[36]

As to micronutrients, 34% of the pregnant women whom they studied in 1994 had moderate to severe anemia (<9g/dl).[37] However, another study reported that 19% of adolescent schoolgirls were anemic (<12g/dl), with another 25% borderline anemic (12–13g/dl). Long-term iron-folate treatment proved to be an effective remedy.[38]

Another micronutrient, iodine, is conspicuously lacking in most inland Sarawak environments. Even today some adults in areas such as the upper Rejang and Lemanak have goiters. Iodized salt and iodated water supplies have alleviated much but not all of this problem. In contrast, mineral springs in the highlands have long been used to prepare iodine-laced salt, which was widely traded among groups in the past.

In all, the many faces of malnutrition are fundamental problems in Sarawak.

---

[30] In 2000, childhood malnutrition in Song District was 37%, in Kapit District 36%, in Kanowit District 25%, and in Belaga District 36% (Anonymous 2000c).

[31] Benster and Stanton 1989.

[32] Yap 1985.

[33] Wee et al. 1996.

[34] E. Garit 2001, personal communication.

[35] Duffield and Strickland 1999.

[36] O'Hanlon 1985.

[37] Duffield and Strickland 1999.

[38] Tee et al. 1999.

Dimensions of Malnutrition

So what are the facts about malnutrition in Sarawak? They are well documented for people who attend motherhood health clinics—that is, pregnant women and small children. They are hardly documented at all for other women, for men, and for adolescents. By all accounts, there are pockets, or perhaps expanses, of childhood undernutrition, mostly in poor families in degraded environments. In contrast, Iban in "suburban" Bawang Assan near Sibu say they now eat more meat than previously was the case.[39]

With Malaysian culture now emphasizing a cash economy, buying food has become the norm. A family has three food options: producing enough food to sustain itself, buying food to achieve that end, or becoming malnourished. Many factors enter into this situation, including government policies, the timber industry, agrobusiness, short fallow periods for rice farming, world market forces, family cash-cropping, and off-farm employment. Often food security is lost in this welter of factors.

Fewer types of foods are now eaten than formerly and, in fact, diets have generally become rather uniform. In the 1970s Engkari and Bintulu Iban farmers grew 27 secondary food crops in their swiddens, plus tobacco and tuba.[40] Kejaman longhouses, above Belaga on the Rejang, grew at least 20 secondary crops in swiddens, plus six kinds of fruit trees.[41] In the 1990s Bidayuh in Gayu village grew 34 secondary crops in their swiddens, with vegetable intercropping being common.[42] However, even if intercropping were common throughout Sarawak, it provided nutritious vegetables for home consumption just for part of the year. Only when people had access to fallow fields and forests were they able to forage for food (and medicinal) plants year-round. With deforestation and giant plantation schemes, this is no longer the case in many areas. While there are many causes of food deficiency, it has received too little attention from the government. To lessen this problem in some areas, kitchen or neighborhood-community gardens could be encouraged and vegetable seeds provided.[43]

Some Sarawak men may not be aware of nutritional issues.[44] When a university student group studying malnutrition in a Bidayuh village near Tebedu reported their findings and advice to the village development committee, a group of about fifteen men, the men heard the students out, thanked them, and said they would work on the students' proposals. One observer surmised that the committeemen were thinking: "Of course the

---

[39] Edwards 2000.
[40] Padoch 1982.
[41] Strickland 1986.
[42] Gerrits1994.
[43] Alexander and Alexander 1993.
[44] In 1950 a father in the modern mode had his newborn fed condensed milk; it died three months later (Geddes 1954).

kids are skinny. So were we when we were their age. So why all this fuss?" Some Sarawak men are even said to think that malnutrition only refers to the plight of the starving Africans they see on television!

Most rural children, once past infancy, look skinny to a non-Malaysian observer. Even educated Sarawak adults have difficulty recognizing stunted grown—the result of chronic undernutrition. After I photographed a skinny Melanau child in Badong village, I showed the snapshot to some Sarawakian coworkers and asked how old they thought she was. No one guessed she was six, as indeed she was. Most of them thought she was four years old. Unfortunately, I didn't photograph the girl's mother who was, if anything, thinner than her daughter and already, in her twenties, missing some teeth. Nor did I get a chance to photograph the skinny grandmother bicycling past on Badong's dirt road, wearing a saucy straw hat and beaming at the world with only four front teeth left in her pink gums.

Childhood malnutrition is recorded in health clinic data. For example, children under seven years of age were studied in 1998 in rural areas of western Sarawak, as were those living in government quarters (GQ) in towns. Some results for moderate plus severe undernutrition, based on weight for age, are as follows:[45]

Lundu GQ	8%
Lundu Bidayuh	23% (average for 24 villages)
Lundu Iban	27% (average for 12 villages)
Semantan GQ	10%
Semantan Bidayuh	43% (average for 10 villages)
Tebakang clinic area	12% (Bidayuh, others)

One remote Bidayuh village, Biawak, had 60% undernutrition for this age group (even though it had a vegetable garden by the preschool and still had forested areas around it).

Childhood malnutrition in Sarawak starts about the time children are weaned, generally beyond 6 months of age. In one study, 65% of rural mothers who had infants at least 6 months old went off to do farm work, most of them leaving their infant at home in the care of a grandmother or other relative.[46] Only 38% of the malnourished infants were looked after by their mother, either at the farm itself or at home. Infants under their

---

[45] Ramah Bt. Sait (1999) personal communication; S. Malong (1999) personal communication.

[46] Hardin and Kiyu 1991. However, one Bidayuh mother worried that if children are cared for by others, "You don't know…whether they have eaten or not" (Hew 1999:110). In the Lubok Antu area in 2000, nurses told me that Iban mothers there still observe taboos on weaning foods, using mainly rice. Also, mothers "go back to the field" when children are a year old; childhood nutrition then suffers. An unusual comment I got elsewhere was that mothers are lazy, uncaring, and busy.

mothers' care were much less likely to be malnourished than those cared for by others, suggesting that nutritional education needed to be given not just to the mothers in a clinic setting but to entire families in their homes. However, this change by itself will not cure malnutrition as other factors intervene, such as low birth weight, low socioeconomic status, and chronic infections.[47]

Childhood nutrition can be helped by providing a free lunch at school. While some kindergartens and primary schools may provide lunch, not all of them in Bidayuh areas did so in 1990 because subsides for the meals were scanty or nonexistent.[48]

The explanations I heard for childhood malnutrition in Sarawak were quite varied: children preferred snack foods to balanced meals; they were not fed properly when their mothers were working elsewhere; wild foods such as meat and fish were no longer available to give to them; and, traditional weaning foods are not nutritious. All these explanations are probably valid.

Childhood malnutrition has lasting effects, visible in older people. Fewer people in Sarawak than in Japan or Europe live to be 60 years old. Many of the elderly people in Sarawak are quite frail. Lack of food security during their lifetime is one reason for this. Infancy and childhood during the Japanese occupation and its unsettled aftermath in the 1950s had a negative effect with repercussions that lasted for many years. But even a few bad rice harvests, some due to El Nino conditions, can be damaging for long-term health.

The hard work of farm life is another reason for thinness in the elderly. This is especially true for women farmers. Also, women who have had many pregnancies are prone to "reproductive depletion," as it's called. Both hard work and pregnancies lead to thinness and weakness. Anemia, for instance, can complicate not only the pregnancies but can weaken a woman's ability to do manual labor in the farm field.

Thinness can also have a cultural basis. Elderly women, in particular, are regarded by some Bornean groups as not doing any real work. Babysitting, mat and basketry making, weaving beautiful cloths, being knowledgeable about herbal remedies, raising chickens, and so on, are not considered work because they bring in little or no money. Consequently these women may not be encouraged to eat well. They might even *decline* to eat well, so as to provide larger portions of meals to younger people in the household. If so, this has implications for now and for the future, because lifespans are lengthening in Sarawak, as in many other places. The number of older people is gradually increasing. While this trend will provide more babysitters for communities, if good nutrition for the elderly is largely neglected for cultural or economic reasons, there will be more

---

[47] Kiyu et al. 1991.

[48] Yaakub et al. 1993.

geriatric health problems. This will rebound on the younger household members, especially the younger women—the first line of health care in Sarawak. If richer countries are anything to go by, it will also mean increasing hospitalization and medication expense for the elderly, both men and women. Families will have to bear some of this cost and the public health system the rest. Neither the public health system nor most Sarawak families are in a position to shoulder this burden well. The "preventive medicine" of better nutrition for the elderly would help avert a more burdensome social future for the entire state.

I have not seen any research report on the general health of elderly Sarawakians but the rural elderly in West Malaysia have been studied.[49] The apparently healthy Malays studied were found to be financially stressed, poorly educated, and in need of better health services. They had some chronic conditions, such as painful joints, hypertension, and coughs, and about 10% of them couldn't walk well. In addition, about two-thirds had vision or hearing loss, half had a loss of appetite or had sleeping difficulties, and 43% had chewing problems. Men and women in this study had about the same number of chronic conditions. The study showed that hearing aids, spectacles, and dental services are basic needs for the elderly. Poor dentition, in particular, can cause poor nutrition.

Malnutrition makes people of all ages more susceptible to diseases. Malnutrition includes calorie deficiencies but also deficiencies of protein, iron, vitamins, and iodine. Infections can multiply, especially when malnutrition is combined with polluted water supplies.

Malnutrition directly underlies most cases of anemia.[50] Anemia is more common in children, adolescents, and women than in men. Its usual causes are insufficient iron and folic acid and its consequences are fatigue and vulnerability to infections. In adults, work productivity declines with attendant economic loss. Older studies found up to 35% of rural Sarawakians were anemic, but today the prevalence is unknown. One recent study found many people with anemia in the upper Rejang watershed, with more anemia among males than females (29% versus 17%).[51] The reason for this odd finding may be that mothers, but not others, are given iron-folate supplements through health clinics. In support of this conjecture, only 12% of the women aged 31–40 years were anemic while 23% of the men in this age group were. In contrast, in the 11–20 year age group 32% of the females but only 4% of the males were anemic. Looking at older people (over 40 in this case), the study tested 55 women and 83 men, perhaps because women's longevity is less than men's. Notably, there were no women who had reached 70 years but quite a few

---

[49] Shahar et al. 2001.

[50] Inherited thalassemias, which exist in Southeast Asia, also cause anemia, but their incidence in Sarawak has not been reported.

[51] Sagin et al. 2002b.

men in their 70's or 80's. Of the 55 older women, 16% were anemic while 40% of the older men were. This higher rate in men is unusual but may be related to poor nutrition or, as the researchers suggested, to alcoholism (see accompanying box).[52] In any event, these Rejang people have now been moved out of their home areas to make way for the gigantic dam project known as Bakun. This forced change is likely to produce new health problems, but not necessarily cure old ones.

Traditional drinking rituals

A 1960s Peace Corps worker who lived in a Kayan longhouse up the Baram River beyond Long Lama wrote:

> The Kayans were a spiritual people, but they were also rather serious party animals. They had a traditional combo [that] called for chewing betel nut until your lips turned blood red, smoking an unidentifiable herbal product in a jungle cigar, and then drinking a highly potent homemade rice wine called *tuak*...The Kayans, like a tribe of persistent mother hens, would push this combination on every guest, and it was considered extremely bad form to turn down their offering. Accepting their largesse, however, would lead to projectile vomiting...If, after being sick, you continued drinking *tuak* with them, the Kayans considered you a man and, even more important, a friend. The only time the Kayans found my behavior socially unacceptable was once when, after an extended harvest celebration, I accidentally vomited on the chief.[53]

Micronutrients

Southeast Asia has long been an area with high rates of vitamin A deficiency, anemia, and goiter. Micronutrient deficiencies in Malaysia have been recently reviewed.[54] More is known about the situation in West than in East Malaysia. The micronutrient of highest interest is iron, since it is needed to prevent anemia. Anemia is fairly common in all age groups in the country, especially women 18–60 years of age, but also boys and girls under age 13 and adults over age 60. Vitamin deficiencies also occur, but vitamin A deficiency, known to cause blindness in children, has declined over the past generation.[55] Iodine deficiency has also declined nationwide. Less is known about the levels of zinc and folic acid in the population, and baseline surveys are needed for them. On the positive

[52] Some Sarawakians do not think of *tuak* (rice wine) or toddy as alcoholic because they come from natural sources; only beer and whiskey qualify. Drinking *tuak* is acceptable but drinking too much water is unhealthy (P. Lindell, personal communication).

[53] Friedman 2002:245.

[54] Khor 2002.

[55] Along the Tillian River, 2% of Melanau children had xeropthalmia due to vitamin A deficiency in the 1970s (Anderson 1977).

side, Malaysia developed a national plan of action for nutrition in 1995. The micronutrient part of this plan aims to reduce anemia and goiter through various public programs, including food baskets for poor families with underweight children, free school meals for poor children, and health education about nutrition. The importance of breastfeeding is also stressed in this educational effort. The goal is to provide a health safety net, especially for growing children.

Surveys of iodine deficiency (goiter) in Sarawak have been reviewed up into the 1980s.[56] In some areas over 90% of adults tested had goiter, the affliction hitting all cultural groups in the state. Rates in children were generally lower but were still of grave concern.

Some micronutrients were recently studied in school children in Bario.[57] The area has well-known sources of iodine in ground water and soils. Copper, manganese, and selenium levels in serum samples from the children were found to be satisfactory. The natural environment of Bario thus seems to be propitious for healthy child development. This Bario study did not include tests for fluoride or other micronutrients such as vitamins. Fluoride is important for healthy teeth and Sarawak has long fluoridated urban water supplies. However, some geological regions of the world do have adequate fluoride in water sources, and so may some Sarawak areas, as yet undiscovered.

Nutritional deficits were widespread in Entabai Iban in the 1980s.[58] Among the rural households studied, 75% of them ate at least 60% of the necessary amount of calories and almost all households ate enough protein, niacin, and thiamine. If it is somehow possible to accept a 60%-below-par level as being normal, the major deficits then become calcium and riboflavin (both having 69% of households below the 60% cut-off level), iron (44% below the 60% cut-off level), and vitamins A and C (both 37% below the cut-off). However, periods of hunger occurred annually when rice supplies were depleted. Moreover, the protein eaten in Entabai was of low quality. Most of it came from rice, which is low in the essential amino acid, lysine.[59] While legumes such as beans are eaten with rice in many world cultures to "balance" the amino acid intake, beans were not grown in Entabai.

Micronutrient deficits and other problems were evident in the 1990s in Mujat, in Serian District.[60] This Bidayuh farming village had many young parents who had never been to school (35% of the fathers and 51% of the

---

[56] Tee 1993.

[57] Zaleha et al. 2003. One sample of home-made salt tested high in iodine, but earlier work by the Sarawak Health Department found home-made salt from these highlands had insufficient iodine (A. Kiyu, personal communication).

[58] Yap 1985.

[59] Rice also has low iron bioavailability. However, rice is more nutritious than sago or cassava tuber, having 6% protein versus 1% for the latter two (Anderson 1977).

[60] Yap 1998/1999.

mothers). About 84% of these families were poverty-stricken, with 40% being classified as poor (an income of RM 248–495 per month) and 44% as very poor (below RM 248). Villagers were not self-sufficient in rice, the revered staple, having to buy it often. But they rarely bought vegetables, meat, or fruits; these were either grown, foraged locally, or not on the menu. Eighteen percent of the preschool children of the young parents studied had been born with low birth weight (LBW).[61] Among these preschool children, over a third of the boys and almost half of the girls had protein-calorie malnutrition. Higher percentages had stunted growth. Significant deficiencies of calcium and vitamin A intake were found in the children, but vitamin C, thiamine, and riboflavin intake was satisfactory. While the parents' nutrition was not studied, the enveloping situation of poverty and educational handicaps in Mujat suggest to me that the parents of the preschool children, especially the mothers, also were poorly nourished and had their own health problems.

Teeth

Poor teeth are another sign warning of malnutrition. This is especially obvious in older, toothless people. Indeed, toothless elders seem to be rife in Sarawak. According to one Malaysian report, 47% of elderly people surveyed had difficulty in chewing food.[62] A generation ago, T. Oldrey lamented the dreadful state of the teeth in the Punan Busang: all but small children had gross decay and many teeth "had crumbled away to gum level, leaving a few discolored stumps."[63] Even in Sri Aman, which got a fluoridated water supply in 1961, Iban secondary school children there averaged 8 carious teeth each in 1970.[64] In the 1980s, 80% of Sarawak school goers, ages 6–18 years, had caries.[65] Many rural areas may have water supplies poor in fluoride, which prevents tooth decay, but the only report I've seen was on Serian District; fluoride was low there.[66] Taro, grown in Borneo, has been reported to be rich in fluoride, but I have never found any confirmation of this claim.

Dentists are rather rare in Sarawak, with one for about every 16,700 people in 2001. Many are private practitioners in towns who are not visited by poor people because of high fees or transport costs. Most of the 26 government dental clinics are also in towns, and while they have low fees, they are understaffed. These clinics do dental education and some restorative work. However, dental education is common in Sarawak

---

[61] The state average was under 12% LBW by 1988, with Chinese having a lower rate and Iban and Bidayuh higher rates (Yadav 1994).

[62] Sushama 1992.

[63] Oldrey 1972:275.

[64] Yim et al. 1973.

[65] Wong 1992

[66] Anonymous 1975.

schools.[67]

People once brushed their teeth with homemade brushes. Some Bidayuh used a sliver of coconut shell full of bristles.[68] Iban used *biansu* twigs.[69] How effective they were in preventing tooth decay is unknown, but Lahanan adults and children brush their teeth regularly and yet suffer frequent toothaches.[70] They over-consume aspirin or panadol for pain relief. While a local paramedic can extract teeth, restorative treatment by a dentist is virtually unavailable. The craving for store-bought sweets in an otherwise non-sweet diet is also part of the Lahanan problem. The children in Lubok Antu are also heading towards this situation. When I was there, as soon as school was out, they drifted toward the local shops to buy as many sweets as they could afford.

The first doctor to visit longhouses in the Ulu Rejang lamented the tendency in the residents to file and blacken their teeth, or to gold-cap healthy teeth.[71] There are still older people in Sarawak with gold-capped teeth, once considered a prestige item, just like old Chinese water jars. Such beautification became a fad when people sold forest produce in town and, being self-sufficient, spent their unneeded cash for capping in the Chinese fashion. Capping, however, provides a safe haven for bacteria to cause unseen tooth decay or gum disease. Capping was once so popular throughout Southeast Asia that in the 1940s at Yuan Chong on the Mekong River, brigands did not waylay travelers with "Your money or your life," but with "Your teeth—thank you!"[72]

Are Dayaks Obese?

During the 1990s, indigenous groups in Malaysia had more underweight adults than other groups in the country.[73] While more indigenous women than indigenous men were underweight (17% versus 12%), more of the women than the men were overweight (26% versus 20%). This leaves 57% of the indigenous women and 68% of the men in the normal-weight range. However, by age 45, both men and women in the indigenous category were found to be thinner than older people in other groups.

In another study, a sample of older Iban men and women was found to have increased about 4 percentage points in body-fat levels between 1990 and 1996, suggesting a trend.[74] However, during this six-year period,

---

[67] Sarawak Medical and Health Services 1986.

[68] Calder 1954.

[69] Sutlive and Sutlive (2001) show a photograph of these toothbrushes on p. 1989.

[70] Alexander and Alexander 1993.

[71] Chong Chun Hian 1993.

[72] Bradley 1945:96.

[73] Ismail et al. 2002.

[74] Strickland and Duffield 1998.

about 9% of the adults had died, possibly those who were more undernourished than average. In any case, the finding that in 1996 an average Iban man 50 years of age weighed 52 kg. (113 lbs.) and an average Iban woman 48 years of age weighed 48.5 kg. (107 lbs.) hardly suggests obesity.

In related work, a sample of 51 Sarawak Dayak men and women was intensively studied, all being in the normal weight range.[75] The men were found to receive almost 50% more "energy intake" than the women. At the same time, the men were less physically active than the women, due to their high level of unemployment. This finding might suggest that, unless things change, the men are headed for more obesity in the future than the women are.

The Larger Picture

All aspects of nutrition (including the intestinal parasites taken up in the next chapter) have both an ecological and an economic foundation. In terms of ecology, some cultural groups in Sarawak are trying to do "crisis management," such as getting their land rights recognized and stopping the looting of forest resources by outsiders.[76] Displaced communities have members who move out of the resettlement zone and become squatters in towns or even on what was traditionally their own land, such as the area around the Batang Ai reservoir. But even in less stressful situations, people have to deal with three parts of their environment: its physical aspects, other life forms (including germs), and the social realm and its processes. Technological fixes work for some problems, such as nutritional blindness (vitamin A), goiter (iodine), and anemia (iron-folate), but other problems are solvable only by people-first approaches.

Modern medical ideas focus on the physical and biological parts of the environment. Does city water contain enough fluoride to forestall tooth decay? Do people get enough vitamins in their diet? Are mosquitoes transmitting dengue virus in a certain village? Such discrete, scientific questions are useful as part of the health equation. Less scientifically, but more realistically, the question is whether people are leading fulfilling lives—useful to them and their living circle, and with their rightful share of well-being. Well-being comes from respect and enjoyment. Crippled or blind people may be useful to, and respected by, a social group, but they may also be humiliated or shunned. All this implies that health is only one aspect of well-being and that health relies on good social relations. All the vaccines, pills, and bandages in a hospital cannot substitute for these social benefits.

---

[75] Strickland and Duffield 1998.

[76] This problem is discussed in Appell 1995.

CHAPTER FOUR

WORMS, CANCER, AND OTHER ILLS

Worms

Perhaps half the world's people have parasitic infections in their intestines. In Malaysia intestinal worms are common in poor or rural people, especially children. Earlier reports found these infections widespread in Sarawak. More recent reports have been few, mainly on the people of the upper Rejang and Serian areas and those of Bario.[1]

In the upper Rejang area, over 40% of the 330 people studied had intestinal parasites of one kind or another: Trichuris, roundworm (Ascaris), or hookworm. Kayans had the most infections and Penans the least. School-age children had more infections than pre-schoolers. The Rejang area itself had more infections than did the school goers surveyed in Serian District (34%), but rural Serian children had more infections than did their town counterparts. In Bario, 14% of the primary and secondary school children had hookworm, 16% had Ascaris, and some had other parasites; over 60% of the children had at least one kind. Many had two kinds. The semi-annual deworming program for primary students in Bario seems to be less than effective. Also, the secondary students are not dewormed, their school principal told me. She hoped to remedy this.

Many factors determine who gets these nematode parasites and when and where they get them. Factors fostering parasitism include crowding in longhouse areas where latrines are not available or not used, or any place where water supplies are polluted, or where no medical treatment is available. Most of the parasites are transmitted by the fecal-oral route. Hand washing with soap is a "modern" remedy, but soap was also once made locally from forest-found ingredients.

There is concern about these Sarawak findings, even though intestinal worms are not usually life-threatening. Why are these parasites important? The answer is that heavy parasite loads during childhood retard growth, including mental development. Hookworm, in particular, is a well-known

---

[1] Lee et al. 1999, Sagin et al. 2002a, Nor Aza Ahmad et al. 1998.

menace; it can cause anemia at any age. Those Sarawakians who believe that the worms are just a normal part of life could benefit from some rethinking.

Old-fashioned Teamwork Works[2]

In 1910, 40% of school-age children in the southern part of the United States had hookworm. A philanthropist funded a group that mounted a publicity campaign about hookworm and, in some districts, treated 400,000 children with deworming medicine. Local doctors told schools and families with infected children that they had to build latrines (privies). And they did. School attendance then rose sharply. By the time the children became adults, they were earning 45% more than those who were never treated for hookworm. This "experiment" showed the economic importance of a strong public health program coupled with local endeavors. More fundamentally, all are necessary to keep people healthy.

Studies on intestinal parasites are usually confined to children, since they are known to be victims. However, adults have been studied in the upper Rejang area. There, the infection rate was higher in women than men, and almost as high as in children.[3] While 57% of the women were infected, 66% of the children were infected, but only 33% of the men. The study team suggested that women were commonly infected because they were in daily contact with children's feces, given that transmission is usually from child to child by the fecal-oral route, and then from child to mother. Where young children defecate indiscriminately and put contaminated hands or almost anything else into their mouths, transmission is continuous, barring health improvements. Even when efficacious, broad-spectrum anti-worm treatment is provided, re-infection can occur rapidly. Sanitary latrines and health education are therefore a priority to lessen the worm burden in Sarawak.

Most infected women in this Rejang study had Trichuris worms, but a few had roundworms or hookworm. The health effects of these worms include anemia, fatigue, malnutrition, dysentery, and retarded growth. W. R. Geddes noted that a gloomy girl became much gayer "after she had been given a dose of particularly effective worm medicine."[4] One good thing that can be said about intestinal helminths (worms) is that their victims, on a worldwide scale, rarely suffer from allergies.[5]

---

[2] Wessel 2003.
[3] Sagin et al. 2002a.
[4] Geddes 1954:39.
[5] Yazdanbakhsh et al. 2002.

Cancer

A number of people in a Melanau kindred in the Mukah area died of cancer.[6] Two women in the family who were sisters had breast cancer in the 1990s. The first sister refused surgery but accepted non-surgical treatment; the cancer later metastasized and she died. The other sister disclosed her cancer only in a late stage, being afraid to acknowledge it earlier. She received radiotherapy and was still alive in 2001.[7]

As people now live longer lives in Sarawak, cancer is becoming a major health problem. The cancer profile for Malaysia as a whole lists lung cancer as the leading type, at 21% of all certified cancer-related deaths.[8] However, in Sarawak the commonest are cervical, breast, and nasopharyngeal cancer (familiarly, NPC). Both breast cancer and NPC can be diagnosed early and treated effectively but cervical cancer, while detectable by a Pap smear, presents more of a challenge. In Sarawak, many patients with cervical cancer do not seek help until the cancer is in an advanced stage.[9] In fact, people throughout Malaysia tend to delay seeking help for cancer conditions, although cervical cancer may be a special case if modesty about submitting to a Pap-smear test is common.

Cervical cancer has been little reported on in Sarawak but considerable information is available on breast cancer and NPC, although for different reasons. Breast cancer receives attention because of efforts to publicize the fact that early detection is important for successful treatment.[10] Hence, breast self-examination is encouraged, posters and other media discuss its seriousness, and health personnel are on the alert for it.

NPC has received attention because it has long been an enigma in Sarawak and Southeast Asia at large. For unknown reasons, it is more common in some cultural groups than others. In Malaysia it is reported to be more common in Chinese males (15.9 per 100,000) and females (4.1 per 100,000) than in either Malays or Indians.[11] In Sabah it seems to be common in Kadazans. In Sarawak it is common in Chinese but especially in Bidayuh. The age-adjusted rate for NPC in Sarawak is 13.5 per 100,000 population for males and 6.3 per 100,000 for females, but Bidayuh have twice the rate of the Sarawak average, even surpassing all NPC incidences recorded in other countries.[12] NPC generally occurs in people over 20 years of age, with a peak age of diagnosis around 40 years.[13] Various reasons have been suggested for the difference in incidence among cultural groups, such as a genetic predisposition or a diet high in salted,

---

[6] Appleton 2004.
[7] A. Appleton, personal communication.
[8] Lim 2002.
[9] Lim 2002.
[10] Sarawak had 105 breast cancer cases reported in 2000 (Wong 2001).
[11] Lim 2002.
[12] Devi et al. 2004. NPC is rare outside of Southeast Asia.
[13] Tang Tieng Swee, personal communication.

preserved foods such as dried fish. Also, Epstein-Barr virus (EBV) is associated with NPC and is activated by tumor-promoting chemicals in some Southeast Asian medicinal plants. Even then, other exogenous factors may be involved.[14] As to treatment for NPC, radiotherapy and chemotherapy can give a disease-free survival rate of 76%.[15]

Thyroid cancer is almost twice as common in women than men in Sarawak.[16] This fact may be related to the higher prevalence of goiter in women. Also, since some older Sarawakians are betel-chewers, they run the risk of oral lesions; these precancerous states were relatively common in rural Sarawak in the 1990s.[17]

Radiation treatment for cancer is limited to general hospitals but chemotherapy is also given in district hospitals and some clinics. Palliative care for advanced cases is provided in a few places by home-care nursing or hospice care.

Goiter in Children

In a later chapter I discuss goiter in women, because of its high incidence in them, but children are also at risk. Iodine deficiency at the fetal stage and after birth can retard brain development, even causing cretinism in extreme cases.[18] Iodine deficiency and associated goiter in pregnant women can thus have chronic effects on the next generation. During the 1970–1990 period, surveys in Sarawak showed a low goiter prevalence in coastal areas (where iodine-rich seafood is available) but up to 78% goiter prevalence among some children in inland locations. Women of child-bearing age often had even more goiter than did the children. One exceptional coastal community had over a 70% goiter prevalence; this was quite likely due to their cassava-eating habit (especially during the frequent rice shortages) since cassava is a potent goitrogen.

In 1993 neonatal iodine deficiency in Sarawak was discovered to be at the 7.5% level in a general survey. By that time iodized salt was being given out state-wide by government health clinics and by community health volunteers for family usage. A study in the 1990s showed that most people in fact preferred iodized salt. By 1997 iodated water systems were common in inland villages and boarding schools. School children are now surveyed every five years for goiter. The goal of government programs is to eliminate goiter in Sarawak.[19]

---

[14] Norhanom and Yadav 1995.
[15] Prasad et al. 2002.
[16] Kiyu 1985.
[17] Zain et al. 1997.
[18] Kiyu et al. 1998.
[19] Kiyu et al. 1998.

The 1993 survey found low neonatal iodine deficiency in Kuching, a higher level in semi-urban Bau, and a high level in Simunjan, even though this area, on the lower reaches of the Batang Sadong, is close to the sea. As a follow-up, eight-year-old school children in these three locations were later studied for goiter, to see if the neonatal findings applied to an older age group.[20] Mothers of the eight-year-olds were also studied. Despite the fact that over 80% of the 803 children surveyed lived in homes where salt was un-iodized and attended a school that used un-iodized salt in food preparation, only four goiter cases were found, all in girls. Several of the mothers in the study also were goitrous. The study showed that iodine deficiency at birth can be largely overcome as children grow and develop.

Hypertension

It seemed that everywhere I went in Sarawak hypertension was worrying people. Lubok Antu Clinic had over 300 cases. Nearer Sri Aman town there were hundreds more. People buzzed about it in Bario. Mukah had hypertension on the mind. Since blood-pressure readings are easy to do without high-technology equipment, hypertension can be diagnosed more readily than intestinal worms, so its prevalence seems to be a reality. How long hypertension has lurked in Sarawak is hard to say. Most everyone attributes it to junk food, salt intake, and lack of exercise, but there are many hard-working, skinny Sarawakians who have it. Life-style changes seem to be only part of the equation. People are living longer, which is probably another factor.

Natural and Unnatural Disasters

Sarawak is not prone to vulcanism, having no volcanos. Earthquakes are as rare as hail storms. Sarawak is vulnerable to the avian flu virus, via stray migratory birds (or infected people) but has been spared so far. Probably the major natural disasters affecting health on the horizon are related to ENSO, the El Nino Southern Oscillation—that is, the years of extreme wetness or dryness due to changes in atmospheric and water circulation in the Pacific. Flooding during torrential rains is no novelty in Sarawak but the severe fires during droughts are a modern development. Recent ones in Kalimantan have caused respiratory distress in Sarawak and elsewhere. These fires are the result of policy failures that foster forest exploitation and land conversion. The 1997 fires destroyed over 5.3 million hectares of forest in East Kalimantan alone. While ENSO was involved, much of the burning was deliberate. The cost of these fires was at least US $10 billion in terms of burned timber, lost tourism revenue,

---

[20] Low et al. 2002.

and ill health in Southeast Asia.[21] Sarawak and other areas were engulfed in smoke from the fires.

Deliberate burning in Sarawak, as occurs during dry seasons to prepare vast oil-palm plantations, also causes widespread respiratory problems.[22] If these fires escape into surrounding forests, especially peat swamp forests, they can be much worse. Although respiratory distress is the immediate effect, the major long-range effect is loss of a sustainable environment.

In general, anthropogenic climate change, resulting ultimately from carbon dioxide emissions and tropical deforestation, is predicted to decrease rainfall, increase temperatures, and accentuate seasonality in places like Sarawak. Continuing droughts will produce more fire-prone areas and Sarawak's coastal plain will gradually flood as sea levels rise.

---

[21] MacKinnon 2005.

[22] Cardiorespiratory hospital admissions increased during the fire-smoke period, especially for people over 65 years of age who had pre-existing respiratory ailments (Mott et al. 2005).

CHAPTER FIVE

WOMEN'S HEALTH

When Margaret Brooke first arrived in Kuching, she asked, "Where are the women?" She was met by a few English women and many Sarawak men, but she meant the Sarawak women. Soon, however, she was happily among the women and came to think of herself as being part Dayak and part Malay.[1] The English men of this private colony did not think of themselves in a similar way.

In West Malaysia there are no village headwomen, as far as the government knows. Villages have male heads. But I heard that in Sarawak some Iban longhouses have headwomen.[2] Although I asked about them when traveling around the state, I never managed to meet with one. If I had, maybe I would have found a leader especially knowledgeable about, and interested in, women's health issues. The village leaders I met were all men and all different. One Bidayuh leader was a government employee who commuted to work, being out of the village from dawn to dusk. An Iban leader I met commuted the other way: he stayed at his upriver longhouse weekdays and went home to his house and family in Sri Aman town on weekends. In contrast, a Kelabit leader I met both lived and worked in Bario, his home turf. (Commuting in and out of remote Bario would be no easy feat!) The point of all this is that women tend to stay at home more than men do, and thus a village headwoman who was anchored at home would likely be more cognizant both of general health issues and women's health issues locally.

Women's health is a different story from that of men in many ways. It's easy to think of women as being more vulnerable to domestic abuse, prostitute abuse, and even general invisibility in social, economic, and

---

[1] Brooke 1986:11.

[2] Jensen (1974) mentioned one Iban headwoman a generation ago. Women have also led other Sarawak communities. Two Kayan women were leaders in the nineteenth century (Brooke 1986).

political terms.[3] This invisibility contributes to less awareness about the health of women than men, whether in the household, the community, or at the national level. For this reason, women's health deserves special attention, beyond important considerations of health for everyone.

In the pre-colonial era when institutionalized authority was minimal in Sarawak, individuals enjoyed a certain autonomy. With such autonomy, one usually finds gender equity. While most major bureaucracies are male-dominated, many village societies in Sarawak were not. The moral and social universe of meanings applied to all—children, men, and women.

However, gender inequality on health care has persisted from the colonial into the present era. Formerly, reproductive issues and maternal deaths were considered the measures of women's health. Now the holistic concept of women's health includes health in terms of work and sexuality. The concept also extends to mental health and issues affecting different age groups. Despite this conceptual improvement, information is sketchy in Sarawak on the range of women's experiences of health versus illness, other than those related to procreation.

Although few health studies exist on Sarawak women, it is clear that their health is better than for women in many other regional situations. For example, Sarawak's maternal death rate in the 1990s was only 7% of that of Laos, 47 vs. 653 deaths per 100,000 live births.[4] The Sarawak rate has fallen even further over the past decade, and the lifespan is increasing.[5] One reason for the good-health situation in Sarawak is that it is not as poor as some nearby nation-states. It is also not overpopulated, as Java is, and it is far from war zones. But Sarawak is not isolated and its health problems may grow, despite dedicated efforts to solve them. Among other problems, Sarawak has environmental degradation, inequalities in wealth and education for men and women, and a sex sector—all impinging on women's health.

Most Sarawak women today look healthy. According to Sarawak Health Department discharged-patient data, women seem to have fewer medical conditions, outside of those related to maternity, than men do. For the record, medically-discharged women have less intestinal disease,

---

[3] For one thing, women lag in education. Among Batang Ai resettlement women 80% had never been to school (Hew and Kedit 1987). See also Yap 1998–1999, on rural Bidayuh.

[4] Ireson-Dolittle and Moreno-Black 2003.

[5] According to Abu Bakar Suleiman et al. (1999), 20% of maternal deaths in Malaysia in the early 1990s had associated anemia. The highest risk groups for maternal deaths were women over 35 years of age, followed by women having five or more pregnancies. Women giving birth at home also had an above-average risk. Theoretically, over 52% of maternal deaths would not have occurred if their health care had been flawless. Geographical remoteness and patient non-compliance with medical advice during pregnancy (such as refusing hospital care) also contribute to maternal mortality. Better education of medical staff was recommended to reduce mortality, especially that due to hypertension during pregnancy and to postpartum hemorrhage, and especially for young, inexperienced doctors.

tuberculosis, viral diseases, gastrointestinal infections, immune disorders, heart disease, respiratory disease, urinary track infections, fractures, or wounds than men do.[6] One nagging question is whether women go to health facilities less readily than men do when they have a problem. While more women than men are listed in outpatient records, are these female visits mainly about pregnancy-related matters or about general complaints?

Still, too many women are malnourished, anemic, overworked, goitrous or victims of intestinal parasites. These and other disorders affect their viability.

Survival and Lifespan

While the maternal mortality for Sarawak in the 1990s was 47 per 100,000 live births, the rate for *indigenous* groups tallied for West Malaysia plus Sabah and Sarawak (East Malaysia) was 92.5, with most of this population being on the Borneo side.[7] Malays, Indians, and Chinese had very low rates. In earlier decades, Sarawak indigenous women were known to die off earlier than men.[8] Some Bidayuh men buried one wife after another. The poor survivorship of Bidayuh women was partly due to the fact that they did more work than men and partly to multiple pregnancies (reproductive depletion). Even in the 1970s the prenatal and postnatal diet for Iban women was maladaptive.[9] Women avoided animal protein during pregnancy. For weeks after delivery, a third of the women ate only rice and salt and for several months many vegetables and fruits were shunned.

Now, however, with childhood mortality declining and contraceptives widely available, family sizes are becoming smaller. The Sarawak maternal mortality rate in 2004 was 20 per 100,000 live births.[10] Women are now surviving longer.

Rural Women's Health: Workload, Migration Effects, Living Conditions

Women have been industrious workers in Sarawak for a long time. Alfred Wallace noticed this in the 1850s. One afternoon in the Bidayuh village of Borotoi, he found many of the men at home, but their wives were still working in the hill fields.[11] Their labor provided two crops a year, one of rice and the other of sugarcane, maize, and vegetables. Later,

---

[6] Khoo Khay Jin, personal communication.

[7] R. Jegasothy (personal communication) provided the indigenous data.

[8] Leete and Kwok 1986.

[9] Anderson 1981.

[10] A. Kiyu, personal communication.

[11] Wallace 1962:53.

at Peningau, Wallace observed that because the Bidayuh villages were high in the hills and the rice fields were on the plains, the people went up and down constantly, much of the way by notched-log ladders because of the steep terrain: "The result is an enormous development of the leg. The women, especially, have most disproportionate calves...by no means improving their appearance."[12] Victorian ideas of female beauty aside, Wallace did sympathize with the women. While he considered Bidayuh to be remarkably free of disease, he thought Bidayuh fertility was relatively low because of "the fatiguing occupations to which the women were subjected."[13]

One hundred and fifty years after Alfred Wallace's visit to Sarawak, I also saw Bidayuh women hard at work. Moreover, most of them had to walk a long way from their home to their farm fields. In Serian District just before dusk, one could see couples trudging home for long distances next to the roads. The men would not be carrying anything but the women would be shouldering a full backbasket of firewood or farm produce. Some women spend 90 hours a year transporting such loads on foot.[14] Because of farm work, Bidayuh villages in Serian District can look like "ghost towns" during the day, as many have noted.

Good health is basic to productive work. In the egalitarian cultures of Sarawak, men and women are complementary and interdependent. From the men's point of view, since women are equal partners, much of the farm work can be left to them. It is merely one part of their unpaid family labor. Men typically left home after crops were planted, not returning till harvest time, partly to avoid the job of weeding the fields.

Traditionally, farm work was a sociable occupation, not regimented to a factory-like schedule. While agriculture may be the best culture, as one Bidayuh man said, farm work can be hot, hard, and tedious. Many Iban women have said that when their family men were away, they were left with all the farm work and became fatigued and ill. Children's illnesses added to their problems.[15] However, while women were the "breadwinners" in a third of the Selako households in the 1970s, only about half of these women-supported families resulted from men migrating out to live and work elsewhere.[16]

---

[12] Wallace 1855:366.

[13] Wallace 1857:205.

[14] Windle and Cramb 1999. In 1971, fifteen Bidayuh women surveyed by Grijpstra (1976) spent 57% of their waking hours farming and 27% housekeeping. This left them with less "spare" time than the men. The women spent over sixty hours per week in farming. Kelabit women in Bario also do most of the farm work (Hew and Sharifah 1998). The same is true for Lanahan women (Alexander and Alexander 2003).

[15] Kedit 1991.

[16] Schneider 1978. Also, Selako women own their family's dwelling and the family's rice harvest.

Many older women stay active and useful as long as possible. Even those over 60 continue to farm to this day; this is the case among the Bidayuh and Kelabit and probably among other rural groups as well.[17] Two Kelabit women gave me a Kelabit name, Dayang Matarih, which they said meant grandmother, but I later heard that this name refers to someone in the old days who flew around and had wings, so I'm a bit puzzled about this agile grandmother.

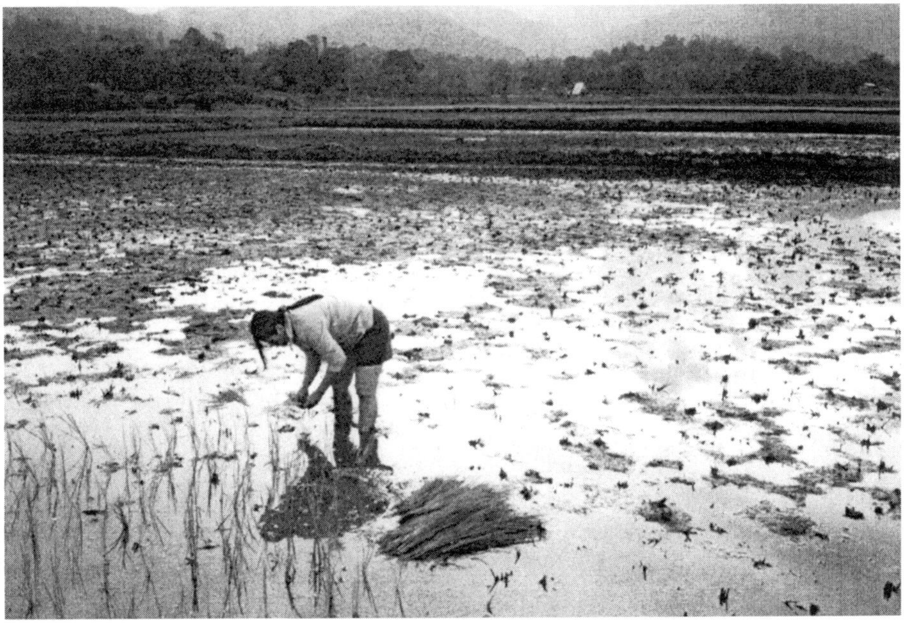

Photograph 8. Rose Tagong transplanting rice, Bario, 2001. Many women are farmers in Sarawak.

Older women work slowly but steadily in the fields, as long as they are able to trek to and from the countryside. The burden of work on both middle-aged and older farm women today is related to the fact that children are now largely in school and young adults depart for advanced study or jobs in cities.[18] Moreover, once children are in school and their mothers accept contraception, either the Pill or tubal ligation, they become "available" for year-round work, often in pepper gardening. In contrast, farming for home consumption once had a slack period of several months

[17] Older Kelabit women, with their detailed knowledge of the landscape, also take younger ones out for a day of net fishing or to collect forest foods and basket-making materials (Bulan 2003).

[18] However, in Limbang District, Iban and Lun Bawang women whose husbands worked elsewhere found they needed to rely on child labor in farming, despite the state requirement that children attend school (Heyser 1995).

for resting up and social occasions. That period presumably meant less work and more enjoyment for the women and their families. That is, there may be less reproductive depletion but more work depletion for rural women now. To avoid this hard work, younger women flock to urban areas.[19] An added problem is that men are considered the "real" farmers in government circles, and women are not given their just recognition in this regard. Farm women may learn about new crops and farm inputs second or third hand.

In both rural and urban settings, men and children depend on women for their daily needs. In addition to a woman's routine tasks, nursing the sick or disabled, including grandparents, can place an extra burden on her. In this regard, it is noteworthy that Iban men in Song and Kanowit had more health complaints than the women did.[20] This health care that women provide to their families, both preventive and curative, is largely ignored by officialdom.[21]

In like vein, Iban traditional healing practices have become male-dominated. Whereas both women and men were once healers (*manang*), Iban women are now being denied "their pivotal role as carers most intimately associated with the physical, emotional, and mental suffering of afflicted community members."[22] Curiously, Iban traditionally had no designated midwives although elder women did help in deliveries.

Environmental Degradation

Most people in Sarawak today either live in a village or are connected to the world of forest and field by family ties or recent memories. About 80% of Sarawak land was once hill forest, containing a wealth of animal and plant life that sustained human culture and existence. But no longer. Politicians' pronouncements about preserving the rainforest and biodiversity have not prevented some city people from becoming wealthy from timber extraction.[23]

The major environmental problems that affect women's health are pollution of land and water resources, soil erosion from several causes,

[19] In a longhouse study in 1996, 30% of the young Iban women (18–30 years old) were living temporarily in urban areas, as housewives, waitresses, or in other jobs. The percentage of these out-migrants declined with age (Duffield and Strickland 1999).

[20] Strickland and Ulijaszek 1992.

[21] For instance, in one case an elderly woman with Parkinson's disease was cared for by her son's wife. And in Batu 15 Village, near Kuching, only women attend meetings about cleaning the village or attend PTA meetings about school issues (K. Edwards, personal communication).

[22] Harris 2001:133. Also among Bidayuh, both men and women were healers, or "shaman elders." They also functioned as protectors and civil-dispute mediators. Every village had at least one traditional midwife, a woman (Schneider 1978). Only female healers performed the *Ngirarang* and *Mgimongi* curing rites (Nissom and Schmidt 1967).

[23] Colchester 1989.

and dwindling land available for subsistence because of the expansion of cash crop agriculture, whether in a huge oil palm plantation or a family plot dedicated to growing pepper or cocoa. With erosion widespread and ongoing, there is a possibility that Sarawak will become a barren land.[24]

Commercial destruction of natural resources impacts women's lives and health. Logging can kill more trees than loggers harvest, and it erodes soils, causes silting, and precipitates flash floods.[25] Aquatic resources of fish, snails, and turtles suffer greatly, not only from turbidity but also from diesel oil pollution. Deer and wild pigs, traditional sources of necessary protein, are now extinct over wide areas. Cash earned from the sale of foraged illipe nuts, resins, herbs, and bamboo has declined. Such foraging no longer functions as a fall-back source of rural cash for buying necessities.

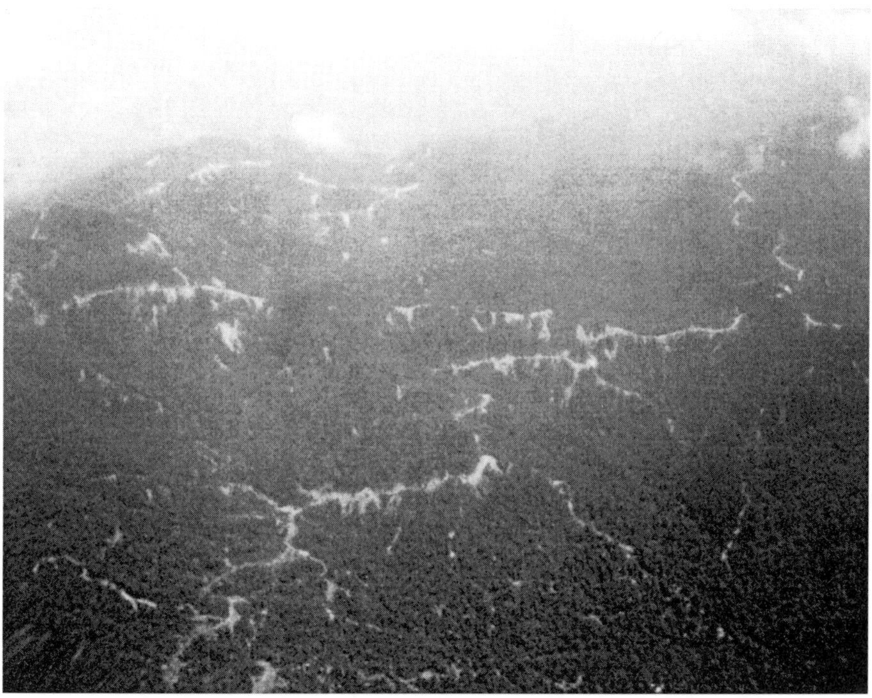

Photograph 9. Logging tracks in the highlands, 2001.

[24] However, I noticed a legume ground cover in a pepper garden just outside Lubok Antu in 2000; it provides fertilizer and thwarts erosion.
[25] WWF (Malaysia) 1985.

While women do not incur chainsaw accidents, as men do, women seem to bear the brunt of the timber and plantation industries' ill effects on health, either directly or in terms of their family. In traditional areas, women collected fern tips and other wild foods in forests and fallows at least weekly.[26] In un-deforested Nanga Sumpa in the 1990s, 103 edible wild plant species were being foraged by Iban, while in Kelabit country, at Pa Dalih, 68 wild species were foraged.[27] In both cases, the menu for meals was far more varied than anything a city restaurant can offer.

Many villages now have tap water, which frees women from hauling water home every day. But the tap sometimes runs dry. The women then have to go back to traditional methods of water collection—from springs, rivers, or swamps—even if they are polluted. In Serikin, in Bau District, some urban visitors complained they could not take a bath when the tap ran dry, but the difficulty of getting water for other household use was not reported.[28] And pour-flush toilets don't work without water.

In the past, all farming in Sarawak was organic farming, with no manufactured fertilizers or pesticides in use. Fertilizer meant the ash layer produced by field burns, the bran produced by hand milling rice, nutrient-laden silt flooding a swamp-rice patch, or, in the highlands, the droppings of water buffalo on a fallow rice paddy. As a result, soils and water courses had no chemical pollutants.

Chemical treatments of villages or farm areas are now common.[29] They have health implications. Besides their cost, agrochemicals present ecological problems. For example, fishing declined in Singai as herbicides became widely used in pepper or cocoa plots.[30] Women often take jobs in oil palm plantations because other work is not available to them locally, but these plantations use large amounts of pesticides, injurious to health. If high-risk pesticides such as Paraquat and 2,4,5-T are used in plantations, the workers' health can be jeopardized. Runoff from oil-palm plantations also kills fish in Melanau areas. Such chemicals also can cause health problems for humans. Effluents from oil palm processing plants have made some major rivers unusable for drinking or bathing.[31]

DDT is another chemical treatment. It has been used for decades in Sarawak to ward off mosquitoes. Spraying DDT for many years was probably seen as a least-bad decision, despite increasing reports on its toxicity to animals and people. It did save lives in a malarious

[26] Hew and Kedit 1987. Dyestuffs for weaving are also foraged; Iban women, for example, use *engkudu* tree roots for red coloring (Chalmers 1998).

[27] Christensen 2002. Medicinal plants were also foraged.

[28] Yaakub et al. 1993.

[29] Burgers et al. 1991.

[30] P. Lindell, personal communication.

[31] Colchester 1989.

environment.[32] Unfortunately, it persists in the soil and can become toxically concentrated (through the food chain) in hen's eggs and breast milk. DDT is therefore a health hazard that won't disappear for many years in Sarawak. Now, happily, other methods are used to combat mosquito-borne diseases in Sarawak.

Beyond these situations, the herbicide Roundup was apparently applied to some children's skin in Bario recently, in a futile attempt to cure scabies there.

Nutrition

Over the past century, women's health has been impacted by many social upheavals in Sarawak, from headhunting and slavery to colonial warfare, Japanese domination, and post-war instability. A generation ago, when today's middle-aged women were born, food shortages were common in parts of Sarawak. In the 1970s, 58% of Bidayuh interviewed said their main problem was food insufficiency and another 20% said health was. About 7% of newborns at that time subsequently died.[33] The diet of pregnant and lactating women was particularly poor.[34]

Largely because of such malnutrition in the past, Sarawak women today are generally small, lightweight people. Iban women average 148 cm. in height and 49 kg. in weight. While heights have remained virtually the same for a generation, weights have increased slightly for women. However, older women are a special subset. Fortunately, the health of older women has received some scrutiny in Song and Kanowit Districts. Among Iban women there over 40 years of age, their height was about the same as younger women, but they were much thinner. They exhibited chronic energy deficiency. This scrawniness was accompanied by sundry ailments and rose in frequency with age.[35]

In the 1970s Tebakang Bidayuh men were eating 2000 kcal per day and the women were eating 1700 kcal, neither amount being adequate for an active life.[36] Recently, 27 Sarawak "Dayak" women were studied for food intake versus energy expenditure. They took in 6.6 energy units and expended 8.1 units, giving them a 20% food deficit. They were in "negative energy balance," not eating enough to sustain them. The 24 Dayak men surveyed were eating 9.3 energy units and expending 9.1, thus

---

[32] Aedes mosquitoes that transmit dengue and Mansonia species that transmit filariasis were shown in the 1980s to have developed resistance to DDT in Sarawak (Sarawak Medical and Health Services 1986).

[33] Grijpstra 1976.

[34] Anonymous 1975, Anderson 1977.

[35] These Iban data are from Strickland and Duffield 1997; Strickland and Ulijaszek 1992 1993, 1994.

[36] Strickland 1986.

being energy-balanced. They were also eating 40% more energy food than the women were![37]

Goiter

Words for visible ailments have remained little changed for thousands of years in island Southeast Asia where Western Malayo-Polynesian languages are spoken today. It is easy to observe goiter (Malay, *begok*), ringworm (*kurap*), leucodermia (*panau*), or scabies (*kudis*), and the names for them are ancient.[38] A *begok* may have first meant any swelling of a body part. When coastal people first expanded through island Southeast Asia they would have had little goiter because they ate seafood that is rich in iodine. But when people moved inland on the large landmass of Borneo, they would have become cut off from marine resources. Most such inland areas have little iodine in the soil or water to provide iodine-rich foods. Early trade in sea salt could have moderated the impact of goiter in inland areas, but I know of no evidence for this for Borneo.

Goiter has been common in inland Sarawakians for generations. It is caused by a lack of dietary iodine. Inland people even today may have goiters because they eat little seafood and their physical environment provides little iodine. In addition, poor people eat both the leaves and tubers of cassava, which contain goitrogens. These compounds snatch iodine from its needed role in the thyroid gland. Less damage is done by cassava leaves when they are cooked with dried anchovies; then the iodine in the anchovies helps to counteract the goitrogenic effects of the leaves. This is a common dish in Sarawak.[39] The inland Lun Bawang, Kerayan, Berian, and Kelabit, however, tend to be free of goiter because their local salt supply comes from iodine-laden water laboriously evaporated from hot springs or wells.[40] Groups in the Baram such as the Kayan and Kenyah once traded for this iodized salt from the highlands. The Kenyah even called the Kelabit "people of the salt."[41]

Women are more prone to goiter than are men. Women lose iodine from the body when they provide it to their offspring during pregnancy.[42] In the Rejang region in 1970, 33% of Iban females and 8% of males were

---

[37] Ismail et al. 2002.

[38] Blust 1995.

[39] Even in ritual meals cassava leaves may be served by Baleh Iban, along with rice, chicken, pork, and green beans (Chalmers 1998).

[40] Zaleha et al. 2003, Bulan 2003.

[41] Sellato 1993. The Kelabit water is salty because it occurs in ancient marine sediments; that is, it is sea water, and sea water always contains iodine.

[42] Recently, 7.5 % of Sarawak neonates were found to be iodine-deficient as a result of their mother's low iodine intake (Kiyu et al. 1998). This is significant because a deficit in early life, even a small deficit, can do life-long damage to the brain, depressing mental ability.

goitrous.[43] Goiter increased from age 10 to age 60 and then the prevalence leveled off, with older people having larger goiters. Likewise in the uplands of the Ai River basin, 99% of the population had goiters.[44] As late as 1993 in Lubok Antu District, 75% of women in the Ai area and 49% in the Lemanak area had goiters, despite the fact that iodized salt had been freely distributed by health workers to this area for decades.[45] To correct this situation, iodine was introduced into the piped water supply of certain villages by the health service. Within one year, their goiter prevalence dropped from a range of 49–83% down to 26–47%. By late 1997, 300 Sarawak villages and 40 government boarding schools had been provided with iodinated water supplies.[46] In addition, legislation now requires that salt sold in goiter-prone areas must be iodized. Also, iodized salt continues to be distributed free to villages that need it. Goiter is now on the wane.

Anemia

Anemia, or blood poor in hemoglobin, is usually due to a lack of iron and folate in the diet. Anemia drains strength and energy, especially for women who lose blood through menstruation and delivery. Nurturing the blood supply of their offspring during pregnancy is another challenge for anemic women.

In one study 47% of non-pregnant Iban women were found to be anemic, compared to 40% for the men.[47] Moreover, 44% of 1,408 girls 12 to 17 years of age studied in Samarahan District were anemic, with about half of them moderately to severely affected.[48] After the researchers provided 22 weeks of treatment with iron-folate supplements, almost all the girls were no longer anemic.

Anemia in pregnant women is a major factor leading to fetal loss or low birth weight (LBW) in offspring. Mothers in Lundu Hospital with anemia, hemorrhage, hypertension, or pre-eclampsia had four times more LBW children than mothers without these conditions—45% versus 10% LBW offspring.[49] As is well known, LBW is a main cause of deficiencies in infant growth and survival worldwide.

---

[43] Ogihara et al. 1972a, 1972b.

[44] Maberly and Eastman 1976.

[45] Foo et al. 1994, 1996. If the iodized salt is rock hard, it is not well received, I was told; it has to be pounded to make it fine-grained. And some people said iodized salt tasted bitter to them.

[46] Kiyu et al. 1998.

[47] Strickland and Duffield 1999.

[48] Tee et al. 1999.

[49] Yadav 1994.

Cancer

In Sarawak, thyroid cancer is almost twice as common in women as in men.[50] Breast and cervical cancers may be on the rise in Sarawak since they are rising elsewhere in Southeast Asia. Government data show that 34 women died of breast cancer in Sarawak in 1999.[51] Sarawak seems to have a high rate of breast cancer, with over 230 cases reported every year.[52] A third of these cases are discovered after the cancer has metastasized. That is, women don't go for a checkup or breast examination in a clinic until the situation is dire. In speaking about breast cancer, a ministerial official in Kuching said that some women prefer spending money on cosmetics and clothes rather than on health. This view surely applies more to younger than older women, and to middle-class ones more than poor ones. However, breast cancer typically appears in women 45 to 60 years of age, and is uncommon in young career women in cities.[53] Although breast-cancer awareness campaigns and other attempts at detecting breast cancer in its earliest phase are laudable, such information may not be effective in getting older or rural women to do breast self-examinations or to report a problem early. Fear of treatment may also keep them from seeking help. Some may shun the disfigurement attendant upon breast surgery, but radiation treatment and chemotherapy are additional problems for anyone to contemplate. All this makes for a difficult situation for women, in addition to their other responsibilities. Also, some Melanau women are non-compliant during the Moslem fasting month, refusing to take prescribed medication then.

Other Problems

In the 1970s Iban women who were studied tended to have urinary tract infections.[54] Women had the same general ills as men: viral and bacterial infections, worms, cardiac murmurs, and stomachaches, except that the men rarely had anemia and the women had mild cases. Older Bidayuh women were found to have much higher filariasis rates than younger women.[55] Older Melanau women are known for their diabetes, anemia, and obesity.[56] In Bario, gastritis and hypertension are common, and scoliosis in older women. Older Lanahan have rheumatism and arthritis.[57]

---

[50] Kiyu 1985.

[51] *Yearbook of Statistic, Sarawak* 2003.

[52] Bernama, 24 April, 2004.

[53] However, in Mukah breast cancer may be relatively common in young women (A. Appleton, personal communication).

[54] Maberly and Eastman 1976.

[55] Patau et al. 1981.

[56] J. Wong, personal communication.

[57] Alexander and Alexander 1993.

Malay and "other indigenous" women have more severe hypertension than any other adult groups studied in Malaysia. This problem increases with age; over 40% of such women past 70 years of age have blood pressure above 160/100. These hypertensive frequencies for women were higher than for the elderly men in these two groups.[58] The cause of this high susceptibility in women is unknown.

Women and the Health Services

Women have some particular problems with the government health system in Sarawak. But, in fact, any patient in a Sarawak health facility may not comply with medical staffers' directives for various reasons. For one thing, people often fear being shut away in a hospital under the control of strangers who do incomprehensible tasks, affecting the patient's mind and body. In one case, a Melanau woman with a high risk of birth complications absconded from the Mukah Hospital in the middle of the night with something uneasy on her mind. She made it home to Oya and, by sheer luck, had a normal delivery there.

The health services in Sarawak respond well to acute problems. Chronic problems, however, may require more information being made available, more time and more money spent to provide and maintain a state of health in a patient. Undernutrition is a prime example of a chronic problem for many women. Although health workers do collect data on its extent and severity, at least for children, such data do not in themselves reveal the decisions and actions needed to solve the problem.[59] Even sensing that undernutrition in Sarawak is associated with poverty, poor literacy skills, intestinal parasitism, land loss, and poor work conditions does not provide enough information. Moreover, people in such poverty settings may be aware of their plight but not of the insidious effects of undernutrition—especially for children, women, and the elderly. People may not solve this problem for many reasons. For example, they may face immediate crises that loom larger—such as a leaky roof or debts. At the same time, front-line health workers who recognize the problem cannot solve it solely in the context of medical information and policies. Both groups are "boxed in."

Poor women generally have greater health problems than more prosperous women. Poor Sarawak women, whether urban squatters or upland villagers, also have greater difficulty in accessing medical services, even when roads are nearby.

Although Sarawak has a good network of health facilities in the state, they may be underutilized by women. In the case of pap smears, available throughout Malaysia, only 25% of women have had one, with rural,

---

[58] Lim et al. 2000.

[59] Pellitier 1992.

poorly educated, and single women especially underserved.[60] Women might underutilize health services for several reasons besides difficulty of access. Gender discrimination is one.

While Sarawakians treat doctors with respect, some medical professionals tend to view women as ignorant, especially poor or rural women. In Sarawak, health services for women are primarily focused on maternal-child care, home economics-style nutrition, and fertility control. Generally, women staffers supervise these matters while men handle other types of problems. That is, women are major consumers of health services administered by a male-dominated hierarchy. Since most specialists are men, the more serious a woman's ailment, the more likely she will be treated by a man. Women are therefore at their most vulnerable when dealing with the most powerful physicians.

Another factor that deters women from accessing health services in Sarawak is the lack of privacy during medical exams. Low attendance at clinics and hospitals could be due to avoiding embarrassment rather than an indication of good health. Also, a professional perspective in which women are blamed for their problems can replace gender sensitivity. This can intensify a woman's feeling of inadequacy when she faces male doctors or medical assistants. In addition, Sarawak people are often treated by professionals from a different ethnic group who do not speak their language or understand their culture.[61]

Mothers may also be held accountable if their children have health deficits, such as being underweight for their age. Thus another dose of blame falls on women because fathers are rarely blamed, even though they may be spending money on their own pleasure rather than on family nutrition.

Beyond these considerations, Sarawak women say they don't go to a health facility because they don't think they are sick, or because they are too busy to go, or because they have no one to watch their children if they do choose to go.[62] Some lack transportation money when they are referred to far-away hospitals, especially if several visits are required for a series of treatments. Others have little confidence in modern medicine.

---

[60] Rashidah 1999.

[61] Even though some do speak the local language, their medical language is still based on externally-defined problems, technologies, and logic—the mindset of modernism. While medicine sees health as a natural condition and illness as unnatural, some Borneo societies view illness as part of nature. For them, health is the result of living in a social group, usually a longhouse. Being away from home, being alone, saps health and causes illness (Crain 1991).

[62] Pregnant Iban in Sri Aman District tend to wait until the last minute before showing up at a health clinic for delivery. This includes women expected to have a difficult birth, even though health workers tell these women they should go to Sri Aman Hospital two weeks beforehand.

In view of all this, Sarawak women may try to solve their health problems first by turning to self-medication or to advice from family or friends, but virtually no studies have been done on this issue. Likewise, little is know about the difference between women's views and the government's views of their health problems. Assuming women's values and bureaucratic values differ, much could be gained by officials paying attention to the health situations of women, listening to them rather than "guiding" them.

Health Information/Education

Health education is virtually a top-down exercise anywhere in the world. Officials decide what advice to give out and hope it will be understood and acted upon. They do not usually consult the people about their views. Grijpstra noted in the 1970s that "home demonstrators" from the Department of Agriculture visited Sarawak villages to teach women "how to grow vegetables, new methods of cooking, hygienic measures, etc."[63] This had little impact on the health of the women or their families because the women had little time or energy for these extra tasks. Had the government workers asked the women what their needs were for improving health, more might have been accomplished.

Today many health clinic walls in Sarawak are plastered with Ministry of Health posters to inform people about health issues. Since not a few rural, indigenous women are functionally illiterate, the fact that a poster is in Malay rather than their own language does not affect them.[64] When it comes to women's films on health, however, problems emerge. Some health films depict urban, middle-class women with Western lifestyles discussing urban motherhood problems.[65] Such scenarios bear no relation to the experiences of many rural Sarawak women.

Ironically, while Sarawak women are encouraged to breastfeed their infants, modern views on female modesty have led some young women to forego breastfeeding because they encountered bare-breast taboos earlier at a government boarding school.[66]

In general, if women did receive better health information, the number who think leprosy is caused by "wrong" foods, weakness, or "dirty" blood would probably decline. Those who attribute serious illness to spirits would be able to reconsider their views. Those who think malaria results

---

[63] Grijpstra 1976:149.

[64] In the Batang Ai resettlement area in the 1980s, 80% of the women interviewed had never been to school (Hew and Kedit 1987). Bidayuh adults in the Serian area averaged only 2.2 years of schooling in 1990 (Burgers et al. 1991). Even in 1998, over 40% of the young Bidayuh parents of preschool children in Mujat village had had no formal education (Yap 1998–1999).

[65] Chandler 1989.

[66] Alexander and Alexander 1993.

from eating too much sugarcane might become enamored with mosquito nets. And certain food taboos during and after pregnancy that are maladaptive might disappear.

In addition, health services can be institutionally blind to the fact that poor women's health is associated with poverty. Furnishing pregnant women with multi-vitamin tablets is a stop-gap measure. Longer-term aid would accrue if women had the same job opportunities as men and received equal pay for wage-work with men. "Approved" women's income-generating projects, such as basket-weaving for the tourist trade, do not alleviate women's poverty or marginal status. Such "development" projects treat women's situations superficially. In contrast, one Bario woman I met, who was in the army reserves, has the ambition of parachuting from an airplane. Such intrepid Sarawak women foretell a more fulfilling future for all women in the state.

Conclusion

The Sarawak economy is changing in diverse ways, some of which foster women's health while others do not. Women's health and their cultural position, which are intertwined, seem to be in flux, but improvements are possible. Moreover, the key to health improvement for whole families is the women: their views, their own health status, their environments, and their workloads. Women's views need to be listened to, their health status outside pregnancy studied, and their working environment improved.

CHAPTER SIX

HEALTH SERVICES

The Brooke dynasty took little interest in health work, despite international urging by the Rockefeller Foundation and allied organizations.[1] In 1950, upland Bidayuh in roadless areas "lived and died in their own communities...without the aid of modern medicine," according to W. R. Geddes, a British social scientist.[2] There were two exceptions: a health officer in town had provided Geddes with a medical kit and Christian missionaries brought medicines on their visits to the villages. For the whole Upper Serian District at that time, infant mortality was high, malaria was common, and worm infestations almost universal. Although the population was expanding, epidemics had recently wiped out 20% of the people in some villages. Tuberculosis, dysentery, goiter, and other ailments also occurred. Despite all this, over two-thirds of the people had never consulted any medical person about health problems. The paramedic stationed in Tebakang town had a potential client base of over 12,000 people. Because he could not visit remote areas often, he saw few sick children. The explanation given by some Bidayuh parents was that since country demons tend to injure children, they were averse to letting them spend a night away from home, as would be necessary if they canoed a sick child downriver to Tebakang.[3] Also, sick people did not visit the paramedic if they lacked the 10-cent fee needed during the colonial period. Geddes advocated a short training course for medical aides, especially for training village women.

The British colonial government first sent a doctor to the Ulu Rejang in the 1950s.[4] He, along with a medical aide, found open-sore yaws there that they treated with penicillin. Malaria flourished, made widespread by logging, according to the doctor. Diarrhea, typhoid, and dysentery thrived

---

[1] Heiser 1936.
[2] Geddes 1961:x.
[3] Geddes 1954.
[4] Chong Chun Hian 1993.

without safe water supplies. Infiltrating diseases such as diphtheria, whooping cough, measles, and polio were appearing. Tuberculosis and goiter were evident. Dental health was bad. Venereal diseases, intestinal worms, skin diseases, and other problems also were found. Health in the Ulus was poor and needed government attention. However, many Kelabit received medical attention from British troops from 1945 to 1952. Then a dispensary at Pa Main was opened, staffed by Gerawat Aren, also known as Ngimat Ayu. He was later chosen Kelabit *Penghulu* and today is the *Pemanca* of all the Kelabit.

When Iban became acquainted with modern medicine, they favored injections to cure infectious disease, being impressed by the way penicillin cured yaws.[5] For other maladies they consulted their own healers, *manang*, who understood breaches of social behavior and the spirit world. *Manang*, herbalists, and other healers remain active today but their roles in health services have diminished.

By the 1970s, 10% of Bidayuh villages in Serian District had a mother-child clinic staffed by a trained midwife. While none had a general health clinic, mobile paramedics served some villages. They visited each selected site twice a month. This service was free.[6] In 1975, the health situation in Serian District was still poor, but after that year the health, agriculture, and other departments of the state government concentrated on improving matters. An anti-malnutrition program went into high gear. Fertilizers were provided to increase the yield of hill rice and of vegetables. General hygiene improved. Communal gardening was fostered by providing seeds and technical advice. In 1978, up to 20 lbs. of seeds were provided per village, yielding over 500 lbs. of vegetables for the residents in some cases.[7] Nutritious food baskets were (and still are) provided to severely needy families.[8] At the six primary schools in the Tebakang area, the students were fed one meal a day (at a government cost of 20 cents each). Despite all this help, in the 1980s Serian District was still a priority for improving health because childhood malnutrition remained widespread. Even today problems persist.

Today the main provider of health care for most Sarawakians is the public health service.[9] Private facilities in towns provide some options but these are out of reach to poor people—too far away or too expensive, or both. Government hospitals in the towns are well used by both urban and rural people. Sarawak has 21 of them, with five hospitals providing

---

[5] Jensen 1972/73.

[6] Grijpstra 1976.

[7] Anonymous 1978.

[8] Food baskets contain rice or noodles; dried peas, peanuts, or chick peas; flour; fresh eggs; dried anchovies or tinned sardines; milk powder; cooking oil; sugar; biscuits; and vitamin/iron pills.

[9] See, for example, Kamil Mohamed Ariff and Teng Cheong Lieng 2002; see also http://www.sarawak.health.gov.my/

specialist services: in Kuching, Sibu, Miri, and Bintulu. Specialist services such as glaucoma testing are done both at hospitals and smaller facilities. The latter include over 200 health clinics. In 2001, the doctor to population ratio was 1:2,840 for Sarawak, including non-government physicians.

Many government health services in Sarawak are accepted and appreciated by its citizens. For example, childhood immunizations are widespread and have obviously cut down on illnesses and deaths that formerly victimized families or whole communities. The development of a road system has also provided better access and usage of clinics and hospitals to people living in remote locations. As for health facilities and personnel, they have multiplied throughout the past half century.[10] For example, mobile health teams and the "flying doctor" service regularly visit the Penan, bringing "joy and delight" to them; their sick are treated and medicines are dispensed free of charge.[11]

The Sarawak Health Department has many diligent workers. It is not unknown for a medical assistant to put in a day's work in a clinic and then be up most of the night treating accident victims, such as young men having motorcycle flip-flops.[12] Nurse-midwives can have similar "overtime." If a medical-transport vehicle finds a logging track impossibly muddy after a storm, nurses have to walk a long way to get to their patients waiting for them in Tepoi, high up on the Kalimantan border. Many such instances attest to this praiseworthy dedication.[13]

When the Iban forcibly displaced by a dam project inundating their longhouses were asked about quality-of-life uses in the Batang Ai resettlement scheme, they regarded the health facilities in the scheme better than the health services available at their old longhouse sites.[14] While schools were also seen as better after resettlement, other quality-of-life issues were seen as worse in the new area, including food availability, cash-crop yields, and hunting for game. That is, while formal health services were good in the new area, other aspects of a healthy life were diminished. Local health services can alleviate, but not overcome, the broad effects of government-caused upheavals.

---

[10] Chew 1994.

[11] Hatta Solhee and Langub 1993:244.

[12] Traditional Iban healers and midwives show similar dedication; no matter how hard they have worked all day, their special work can require them to stay up all night (Chalmers 1998).

[13] Calder (1954), for example, lauded the dedication of a medical assistant in charge of a coastal-riverine mobile clinic. He treated over 300 patients per week from his small boat (*perahu*).

[14] Ayob and Yaakub 1991.

Health Provision

The Malaysian government decides the health services its citizens will receive, but these decisions can cause problems of implementation at the local level. In Gayu I heard that improvements health workers suggest in staff meetings often take years to reach fruition. In Mukah and other places I heard that the Ministry of Health (MOH) in Kuala Lumpur micro-managed public health care. There were too many ministerial orders, too many conflicting orders, too much paperwork, and not enough partnership with health workers to plan and implement policies appropriate for the local situation. Generally, the Malaysian government is an over-enthusiastic administrator when it comes to health.

But, according to earlier reports, all this is not new. Dissatisfaction and frustration also affect urban hospitals. A Penang doctor said:

> Political machinery works all the way through the hospital. The hospital is really a government arm. Doctors have to sing to the music of the establishment all the time.[15]

Another hospital doctor said:

> I'll remain voluntarily, to serve the community of people who would not otherwise be able to see a specialist for economic reasons, but only until my frustration with the ways in which the government decides things overcomes my emotional, ethical, and moral desires to serve.[16]

These are strong words and may be deserved in some cases. Historically, Malaysia has followed the government-knows-best mode that British colonial rule bequeathed it. It is not structured for effective decentralization. In the vast rural areas of Sarawak, government deficiencies crop up. In some ways supervision of rural health care is lax, in other ways it is dictatorial. The saving grace for Sarawak is that it is far from Kuala Lumpur, and its State Health Department is thus not under the MOH microscope as much as peninsular institutions.

Still, the paucity of doctors—government or private—in rural Sarawak is obvious. Personal reasons for avoiding such rural work are legion. Private practitioners know that rural people cannot pay as well as urban clients. Any doctor knows that better schooling is available in a city for her or his children. Urban people can find rural settings boring and intellectually isolating. Professional facilities are poorer in rural areas; even telephones, potable water, and electricity supplies can be chancy. Finally, modern-trained medical people may not want to learn the local

[15] Wiebe and Rahim Said 1980:148.
[16] Wiebe and Rahim Said 1980:169.

language and cultural beliefs, and without this knowledge they will be less effective in rural areas.

As far as I know, no one has studied health care facilities and processes in depth on the ground in Sarawak and published a report on their findings. But such a report exists for Sabah. Glen Chandler (1989) studied Keningau and Nabawan/Pensiangan districts, visiting their health facilities and talking with rural Dusun and Murut villagers. She had a lot to say about the district hospital, rural clinics/dispensaries, mobile health clinics, mother-child clinics, and the flying doctor and emergency evacuation services. Being thorough, she also discussed preventive health care in terms of rural sanitation programs, health education, and economic development. She found health care was better in towns than in rural settings and better in some rural areas than others, for several reasons. For rural services, she found that most health workers in her study area served for short periods in different locations on a rotational basis, not permanently in one location and not in their own communities.

Many of these findings also seem to apply to Sarawak. About the inequality among rural areas, a lot depends on the weather and other factors outside of human control. In bad weather, flying doctors cannot fly and boat visits are impossible to coastal areas lacking roads. Generally, the remote communities get "missed" more than suburban ones. Conversely, people in backcountry areas cannot themselves travel to towns for help if they lack money to pay for a long bus ride, they are too ill to travel, rivers are in flood, or the South China Sea is in storm.[17]

About the rotation of rural health workers, this is a good-bad situation in Sarawak. It is good in that people don't fossilize in one place, like the proverbial Malaysian frog living under a half-coconut shell. It also provides an opportunity for people of one ethnic group stationed in another group's area to learn to appreciate the latter's culture. At the same time, rotation can disrupt a medical team's knowledge of local patients and their problems or foibles. It can also be hard on the worker's family to be moved around, in terms of schooling and other considerations.

In Sarawak there are both stationary clinics and mobile clinics, at least in some areas. Mobile clinics try to keep to a strict schedule, but inclement weather and transport breakdowns hamper this. When people trek to the meeting spot from surrounding areas for the expected arrival of the mobile clinic and it does not show up, not only are would-be patients not helped but local work patterns are disrupted. During critical phases of the farm cycle, this can be more than annoying. Fortunately, mobile health teams that visit some remote villages stay over night there. This means that people who could not meet the team at a specific time of day because of some problem can access it over a longer period. It also means that the

---

[17] People in the Iban longhouse of Ensika can access the nearest clinic (at Pekan Sebangan) only during high tide by an hour's boat ride (Andrew and Wong 2000).

team gets to know the community's problems better than if they rushed away quickly.

I do not know if the policy of dispensing drugs by medical clinics is as liberal in Sarawak as it was earlier reported it to be in rural Sabah.[18] There, villagers were given whatever medications they asked for, including antibiotics—even if there was no evidence that an antibiotic was needed. If this is true in Sarawak, it deserves a re-appraisal because of the worldwide increase in antibiotic-resistant bugs that can incapacitate and kill people. Over-prescribing antibiotics and their casual over-usage are harmful in the long run. And yet, many antibiotics—such as those used to treat stomach upsets—are readily available in Malaysia at many chemist shops for self-administration. Likewise, if anti-malarial drugs are available, over-usage or inappropriate usage can occur. For anti-malarials, this leads to drug resistance in the malarial parasite, making this widespread menace harder to cure over time. That is, the effect of impulsive self-medication is cumulative and insidious: the bugs and germs become better and better invaders of the human body.

I also do not know of any reports on the general effectiveness of the flying-doctor service in Sarawak today.[19] At least in the 1980s this service, out of Belaga to upriver longhouses, was cut from once a month to once every six weeks because of government economies.[20] The flying service is greatly at the whim of the weather, especially during the monsoon season, and people can wait in vain for a flying doctor or nurse to drop out of the sky. In the 1970s a Chinese woman doctor and three nurses visited Lusong above the Bakun rapids after a six-months absence but stopped there only for 25 minutes.[21] For various landing fields in the Kelabit Highlands, and probably elsewhere, the unpredictability of visits is true not only for the flying doctor but for emergency airlifts to a hospital or clinic. Even upon arriving at a remote location, a flying medic may find no electricity, no radio contact, and no working telephone, among other impediments to performing his or her duties. Without a telephone or radio contact any health worker or patient has problems consulting with a specialist back at the hospital or making a necessary appointment for a hospital visit.

A particular problem for a male doctor can be a social taboo against him being alone with a woman patient in a private room, let alone for him to do a pelvic examination or any pregnancy-related physical exam.[22] However, I did meet one male obstetrician in Sarawak who maintained that he encountered no such social problem. And while the majority of

---

[18] Chandler 1989.

[19] A flying team usually consists of a doctor, medical assistant and two nurses (Kamil Mohamed Ariff and Teng Chong Lieng 2002).

[20] O'Hanlon 1985. Heyser (1995) reported that upland women thought the flying service was cut to protest the local resistance to massive logging.

[21] Barclay 1980.

[22] Chandler 1989.

older doctors in Sarawak are men, women are quite numerous among the people in medical training now. If these young women follow general trends, many will become obstetricians and gynecologists, allowing their women patients to feel more comfortable in the presence of an examining physician.

When considering emergency evacuations—whether for injuries, complications of pregnancy, or other problems—the major difficulties seem to be weather and human foibles. When I was upstream of the Batang Ai reservoir, where no telephones exist, I heard that to bring a woman nearing a difficult delivery by boat down to the Batang Ai Dam and then by road to Sri Aman hospital could easily take three or four hours. This depended on the up-river starting point, whether a vehicle happened to be at the dam (unlikely in the middle of the night), and other uncertainties. Such delays can be life-threatening. Moreover, I know that in at least one rural clinic, the sole vehicle there for *any* job—including emergency evacuation—was not available when the driver drove it home at night to his house in the town, an hour away from the clinic. Even worse, in a rare incident a hospital driver in Mukah evidently refused to drive an emergency case to Sibu because it was Gawai (festival time).

Dentistry

Dental services are offered in many areas to some extent. About 37% of Malaysian dentists work in the public sector, meaning that almost two-thirds are private practitioners.[23] Sarawak had 81 dentists in 1996, with a dentist to population ratio of 1 per 23,700 population, compared to 1 per 27,000 in 1986, at which time the government service had an acute manpower shortage.[24] In 2001, the ratio was 1:16,700, including those dentists in private practice.

Government dental clinics serve the public, largely in urban areas. Dental officers also visit some rural areas, and in some health clinics medical assistants extract teeth that are acutely painful. Preschool children and antenatal mothers receive some dental treatment and educational materials at maternal-child clinics.

The training of dental nurses started in the early 1960s and by 1992 there were 169 such nurses in Sarawak, giving about one nurse to every 2,000 school children in the school dental service.[25] These nurses give education, extract milk teeth, and clean and fill permanent teeth. In 1992, 192 schools had static dental clinics and mobile clinics brought dental

---

[23] Anonymous 2001b. In Sibu, private clinic patients had, on average, a monthly income two times that of public clinic patients (Chu and Raja Latifah 2001).

[24] Sarawak Medical and Health Services 1986; "WHO Oral Health CountryProfile" 2000, see http://www.whocollab.odont.lu.se/wpro/malaysia/data/malaysiamanpow.html/

[25] Wong 1992. While the Mukah town schools had dental nurses in 2001, I was told that the outlying schools had none, for unknown reasons.

services to outlying schools. Primary school children were given toothbrushes and tubes of fluoridated toothpaste. The dental education at schools includes talks, demonstrations, puppet shows, and poster-design competitions. Today, more than 200 dental nurses staff the school service. This service has long been disease-oriented and less focused on emphasizing early intervention to prevent tooth problems. For example, in one study 30% of the dental nurses questioned did not realize that starting dental education in the youngest school children was more effective in the long run than concentrating on the older students.[26]

In the Kelabit Highlands, a special visit by a dentist was slated to occur the day after I left Bario. This was a welcome development, since a plane trip to a town dentist is expensive for anyone there. I was told that this visiting dentist would only pull out teeth, not do any restorative work.[27] Since Bario has no electric supply except for small generators, this was understandable. (The mini-hydro project for Bario was an expensive flop, maybe not rectified to this very day.) However a Bario school leader was working to provide some restorative dental services in Bario with the help of a city dentist, a Kelabit man, who offered to visit Bario on his own initiative and provide the service for free.

Dentists in Sarawak see "betel chewer's mucosa" in older people as well as oral cancers or precancerous conditions. In one survey oral pre-cancer occurred in 2.5% of the Sarawak and Sabah adults who were studied.[28]

Urban areas in Sarawak have had fluoridated water supplies for over a generation now. This undoubtedly counteracts some of the ill effects of munching on sweets. It may be that some geological features of Sarawak provide useful levels of fluoride in surface or well waters. A map of fluoride distribution in the state would identify such areas.

Health Promoter Volunteers[29]

In 1983 Sarawak introduced the village health promoter program state-wide, later renamed the village health representative program (*Wakil Kesihatan Kampung*). These unpaid representatives, or *wakils*, are men and women selected by their village to provide it with basic health needs. They are supervised by the mobile health teams in their areas. Before the volunteers begin work, they are trained at the areal health clinic (*Klinik Desa*) for three weeks and then given medical kits to take home.[30]

---

[26] Chen and Raja Latifah 2000.

[27] Some medical assistants do extract teeth, but the one stationed in Bario at that time had not taken the training course to qualify for offering this service.

[28] Zain et al. 1997.

[29] This section is based in part on Fauziah Zainal Ehsan and F. Siner Sipeng (1999).

[30] Their training program was considered to be overly didactic in the 1990s (Wong 1996).

Refresher courses are given to them annually. By 2001, over 2,900 *wakils* had been trained, covering more than 1,500 villages.

Besides referring serious problems to their nearest health clinic, the health promoters collect blood slides for malaria and sputum slides for tuberculosis testing, see to trash disposal, and provide treatment for malaria, diarrhea, worms, anemia, conjunctivitis, respiratory problems, skin diseases, and oral conditions. Fevers and coughs top their list of complaints, but worms, headache, diarrhea, skin diseases, and stomachaches are not far behind.

Because of their remote location, mobility and low literacy rate, the Penan of the Baram District received special health-care attention in the 1980s.[31] Their health was compromised by goiter (42% of 395 Penan examined, with women having twice the rate as men), childhood malnutrition, intestinal worms (35% of children studied), dental caries, diarrhea, coughs, and skin diseases such as scabies. To provide basic care to scattered Penan groups, each group agreed to select a husband-wife team to be their *wakils*. To help these teams do diagnoses, a training manual was developed for them that depicted common ailments, along with a text in the Penan language. Clinic and flying-doctor teams oversaw the training and ongoing supervision of the Penan *wakils*.

I do not know the contents of the *wakil* medical kit, but whether a village has a *wakil* or not, all villages, especially remote ones, need medical kits. An example of a list of medical supplies adapted for rural Malaysia is given in the accompanying box.[32] A general set of medicines and their correct usage are described in a well-known handbook on women's health.[33]

---

[31] Chen 1987.
[32] Modified from a list provided by C. Nicholas.
[33] Burns et al. 1997.

Basic Medical Kit for Rural Areas

General per household:
Antiseptic soap
Dried anchovies (*ikan bilis*)
Iodized salt
Toothbrushes and toothpaste
Cough drops

Household or longhouse first-aid kit:
Plasters (adhesive or duct tape)/band-aids (various sizes)
Gauze bandage rolls, 1 to 3 inch
Sterile wound dressings
Alcohol swabs
Cotton wool
Skin closure strips
Liniment/ointment (Vaseline jelly)
Vicks/Tiger Balm
Crepe/woven/elastic bandage
Antihistamine
Antiseptic cream (Savlon/Centrimide)
Eye ointment
Painkillers (Ponstan/ Beafemic 250 mg./Mnefenamic acid)
Diarrhea tablets
Eno sachets (for stomach upsets/heatiness)
Poh-chai pills/*Pil chi kit* (for stomach upsets/diarrhea)
Mentholated oil (*minyak angin*)
Tweezers
Scissors and blade/scalpel
Plastic bags to keep things clean

Bulk purchases for general distribution:
Gastric tablets (Gelusid/Neutrazid)
Antiseptic cream (as above)
Fever tablets/Paracetamol (Panadol/Uphamol 500 mg./Milidon)
Painkillers (as above)
General antibiotics (e.g., ampicillin: Ampicap-T, 250 mg.)
Multivitamins (e.g., Revicon forte 500s, Revicon + iron plus)
Flu tablets (e.g., Beatafed, Decolgen)
Anti-diarrheaic (Loperax, 2 mg.)
Calamine cream
Acriflavine lotion (e.g., Poly Lab)
Cough mixture (Woods, Breacol)
Anti-malarial tablets

CHAPTER SEVEN

PREVENTIVE HEALTH ISSUES: CONVENTIONAL, TRADITIONAL, COOPERATIVE

Modern Methods

Preventive measures carried out by the Sarawak Health Department include vector control, sanitation programs, health education, potable water programs in rural areas (including iodination of water supplies), and school health services. Probably more programs exist than I am aware of. Also, services offered by other government departments affect health, such as advice or seeds or fertilizer from the Agriculture Department that can improve nutrition.

Malaria and mosquito control measures have a long history in Sarawak and have changed drastically over time as malaria became less of a scourge. I have written about malaria elsewhere, as have many other people, and review some of that story in other parts of this text.[1] I'll only mention here that, as for other infectious diseases that have declined, the Health Department must keep a constant lookout for new hotspots of malaria (such as in immigrant workers). Despite the hyperbole in the West that a vaccine is in the cards, malaria will likely persist in Sarawak for years to come. Control measures also exist in Sarawak for diseases such as dengue, filariasis, and cholera, but not even by a leap of faith could one say that measures are in place to control sexually-transmitted diseases such as AIDS.

Sanitation workers pay attention to cleanliness in public situations. In open-air food markets, they monitor both food cleanliness and cleanliness of the food sellers. Sanitation workers are also concerned about contaminated water supplies and many other matters. All this is in aid of minimizing outbreaks of infectious hepatitis, intestinal parasitic diseases such as gastroenteritis or cholera, and so on. But installing water pipes

[1] Baer 1998, 1999a, 1999b, 2003.

from springs, or digging wells in villages that once used fecal-contaminated sources of drinking water, is just a first step to sanitation.

I've noticed that even in public washrooms in cities, soap is seldom used for washing one's hands after using the toilet. I once put a bar of hand soap in a soap-less public washroom for women at UNIMAS, a Sarawak university. I saw many students use the washroom but none used the soap! Yet some women office workers did use the soap. When I asked them why the students did not, an Iban secretary put a polite "spin" on the situation, saying that the students might not want to use someone else's soap. Whether the students really thought that public soap was dirty soap, or that they had no right to use any soap provided, I never managed to find out. A good sociologist of soap could probably answer this question. The end result of my "experiment" was that the bar of soap disappeared. This was a welcome outcome in that I could look on the bright side, believing that someone was so enamored of soap that she had taken it home with her.

American Problems

The American Society of Microbiology reported in 2005 that some people do not wash their hands with soap after using the toilet in public restrooms: 25% of the men observed and 10% of the women did not. Evidently members of this society loiter in public restrooms every year to obtain such data.

Many Southeast Asians don't eat salads, unless they're cooked or the leafy pieces are scalded. The cooked ones can be soupy. So when I was advised in a village to put my market-fresh lettuce in the bubbling soup, I did it. While the soup tasted good, the best benefit of this non-American soup was sterilization of the lettuce leaves. With not enough toilet paper and soap to go around, raw vegetables are only for the daring. The use of chemical fertilizers to replace what the British euphemistically call night soil doesn't change the situation.

Going beyond salad and soap, one problem with piped water supplies is that during a long drought the tap may go dry—even in the fabled monsoon tropics.[2] Or the pipe may get broken or get clogged up with debris. Or the water source may not have ever been large enough to meet the needs of the local population. In a society where the government provides water pipes—or has wells dug—it is easy for villagers to think of these developments as belonging to the government and not something

[2] Water supplies are low in Bario in the dry season. Water-storage tanks are needed for every household but were not common when I was there in 2001. Even the health clinic lacked a water tank although it had requested tanks several times. The large plastic water tank at the airport cost RM 800, I was told, so a fair amount of money is involved in this problem. Bario children were said to get diarrhea in the dry season because of the water shortage.

they should get involved in. In contrast, I've seen places where a village itself installed water pipes made out of split bamboo and, interestingly, these pipes were faithfully maintained.

When Sarawak Health Department professionals surveyed rural water supplies in 1989, they found that a third of the water systems were fully functional, another third were partly functional, and the rest were not working.[3] Through the water-supply program, over 3000 villages had benefitted to some degree by 1987—and undoubtedly many more have benefitted by today. Most of these water systems were gravity-fed, about 20% had rainwater tanks, and the rest had dug wells or other innovations. Because of imperfections in these systems, not as many people were served as these figures suggest. In the 1989 survey, only some 80% of the households had water systems that worked, but some of these (such as rainwater tanks) did not work during the dry season. The survey people recommended that a maintenance system be implemented.

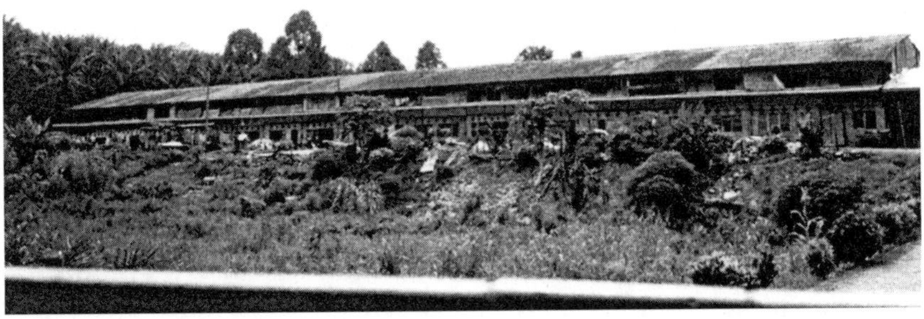

Photograph 10. An Iban longhouse with ornamental plants by the roadway (right) and a trash problem, next to an oil palm plantation, Sri Aman District, 2000.

Another consideration in village sanitation issues involves digging holes and installing pour-flush toilets. When non-health officials come to a village they may inspect it favorably, but I wonder how many inspect the condition of the toilets. These toilets may be dysfunctional (no water in sight) or even unused, especially by barefoot children who are easy

[3] Kiyu and Hardin 1992.

victims of intestinal worms. Even if the toilets are used, a soap-less aftermath is a possibility.

The Truth about Trash

A sure sign of modern ways in rural or squatter areas is trash. People are told it is modern to buy food and supplies, rather than to get them from farms and forests. For a longhouse stuck in an oil palm plantation, there's little space for growing vegetables and no forest convenient for foraging, or for finding timber or bamboo. People also try to be modern by buying gadgets, gizmos, and other ephemera. But where to put the trash? Out the kitchen window, often. There the plastic, tin cans, old batteries, and other junk pile up because they are not biodegradable.

To be more modern would require a rural incinerator or a trash and garbage collection service, just as the towns have. Otherwise, when a city official shows up, the longhouse people may be told to clean up the area, since beautification is considered paramount.[4] However, proper disposal of the trash is more important. Trash provides breeding places for disease-carrying insects and rodents, and old batteries and pesticide containers are not child- or environment-friendly. When city people call villagers dirty because of trash, they forget that they would be just as "dirty" without their urban trash collection services.

Sarawak also has a program of health information. This is quite obvious in the colored posters decorating the walls of health clinics. Some people even call them Ministry of Health publicity posters. For those who can read Malay, the posters give vivid details about examining the breast for cancer, about correct infant nutrition, malaria control measures, tuberculosis, and other official concerns of the day. (If there is a poster on how to avoid sexually-transmitted diseases by using condoms or one condemning male promiscuity, I missed it.)

In addition, published reports detail how demonstrations are given to mothers for preparing nutritious weaning foods, or given to women generally for preparing balanced meals. Reports also mention visits by dental nurses to schools to show children how to brush their teeth and by other professionals on popular health issues. Again posters (or flip charts or pamphlets) are involved. My information about these kinds of health information is largely second hand and thus inadequate to estimate their general effectiveness. But the fact that posters are liberally displayed might suggest to a skeptic that they are the planned endpoint of some health education measures and thus perfunctory. For one thing, I recalled the Iban woman who told me she had a lump on one breast (and had me feel it), but when I mentioned this to a nurse from the nearby clinic when

[4] One official's solution was that anyone not picking up trash should be fined RM 30 (about $9 US), or so he said.

chatting over coffee, she said to tell the woman to come to the clinic and they could refer her to hospital. The woman already knew that, but she probably would have benefitted by a casual, neighborly approach from the nurse since she was frightened of being sent to hospital. That is, health-clinic people in some places could be more "pro-active," to use a catchphrase. On another matter, although there is benefit in instructing school children to brush their teeth, it does not seem to translate into good dental health in Sarawak, as I discussed earlier.

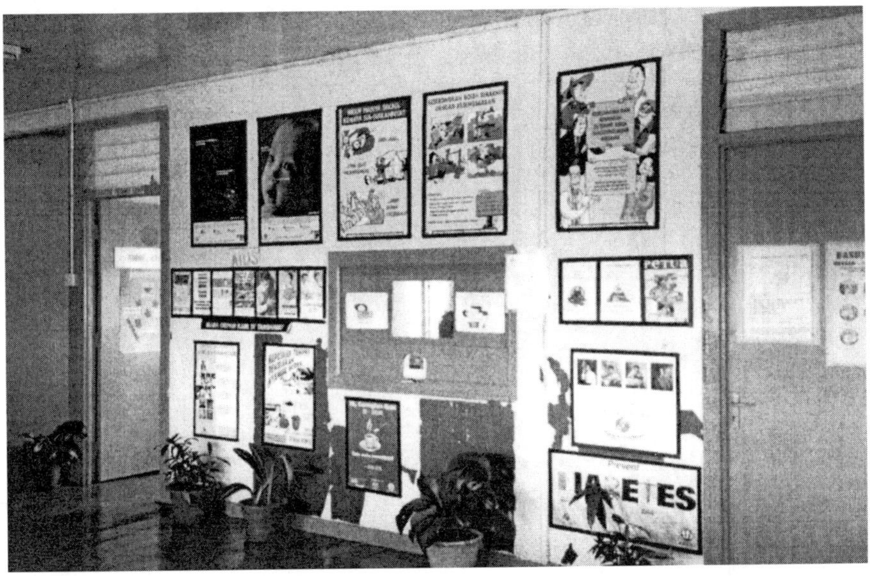

Photograph 11. Health posters at the Bario clinic, 2001. One poster reads "Prevent diabetes" and another warns of the Aedes mosquito. On the left is a panel about AIDS.

Health-clinic people *are* making headway in terms of cancer awareness. Even along the Tinjar River in Baram District in the 1990s, 33% of the women interviewed in one study had heard of self-examination to check for breast cancer and 17% had heard of Pap smears to detect cervical cancer. This knowledge was in great part due to the educational efforts of the health-clinic staff.[5]

In terms of health education about sexually transmitted diseases, it seems that there is no safe-sex education in schools—only so-called moral

[5] Wong and Abdullah Mohammed 1996.

education.[6] The effectiveness of this education is questionable, although perhaps not to the policymakers who instituted the program.

All health-education films emanate from the Ministry of Health in Kuala Lumpur, I was told. This raises another question about their effectiveness when they are shown in rural areas. They may depict prosperous Malaysians in opulent settings, disjunct from the lives of many people; this was the case for a film that discussed combining breastfeeding with city work schedules which was shown in a rural area.[7] As one woman said in another context, "Are they making fun of us?"

If health education were more effective, there might be few cases of non-compliance with medical worker's instructions for patients. Some information from Sabah on tuberculosis patients is relevant on this problem of non-compliance: both compliant and non-compliant patients—for receiving chemotherapy—were interviewed.[8] It turned out in this case, just as for other medical situations, that it cost more, and took more time, for the non-compliant ones to get to the treatment center. Also, the non-compliant people were more apt to have duties that demanded their attention than the compliant ones. Finally, the non-compliant people, when they became free of symptoms, tended erroneously to think that their treatment could be stopped. This last point shows that health education must be ongoing.

In sum, modern health education is well covered in Sarawak, from the school curriculum to the mute posters in health-department settings. There are also government announcements on television and radio, especially when an epidemic looms, such as for Japanese encephalitis. In addition, government personnel visit villages, club meetings, and the like to lecture people about health, as do some non-governmental organizations. Finally, television ads tout the beneficial effects of everything from soap to skin cream.

Traditional Methods

In the nineteenth century, Bidayuh were said to believe that getting wet out in the rain brought on malaria, so they took shelter before the first leaden drop fell or they used Chinese umbrellas, if they had them.[9] This "preventive" measure didn't get to the core of the problem because the rain-mosquito-malaria connection wasn't completely clear to them, or to anyone else in the world at that time. Also at that time, Kenyah erected tall

---

[6] A national women's organization urged the Johor state government to fund safe-sex education. Instead, the state decided to fund HIV testing as a pre-marriage requirement for Muslims (Anonymous 2002).

[7] Chandler 1989.

[8] O'Boyle et al. 2002.

[9] Brooke 1986.

wooden, anthropomorphic statues in front of their longhouses when a cholera epidemic approached.[10]

Among traditional ways of coping with illness, shamanic therapeutic events may be disappearing, without much study of their psychological or sociological efficacy, let alone their ethnomedical value.[11] But other traditional measures remain important today in Sarawak, either locally or more widespread. For example, Iban women avoid sick people in order to guard their health during the risky time of pregnancy.[12] And an obstetrician I met in Daro acknowledged that traditional midwives know how to rotate a breach better than most doctors do.

Medicinal plants have long been used for many preventive and curative ends.[13] Penan in the 1980s knew over thirty plants that were useful for everything from improving a child's appetite to treating coughs, stomachaches, fever, ringworm, headache, toothache, and rheumatism. Five plants were also used as an antidote to dart poisoning.[14] Betel nut chewing is a traditional social pastime, some say a craving while others say an energizer. It is a well-known treatment in tropical Asia against intestinal worms. Betel-blackened teeth also protect against tooth infection.[15] At the same time, betel nut chewing is associated with oral cancer, as I mentioned in an earlier chapter. The health question is one of trade-offs. The social question is one of old versus new ideas, such as cigarette smoking, which raises more health questions. Cigarette smoke is replacing hearth-fire smoke as a lung irritant, because cigarettes are replacing betel chewing and cooking is now often done with gas or electricity. But hearth-smoke can keep mosquitoes (which can carry filariasis, malaria, or virus diseases such as dengue) at bay. Cigarette smoke is ineffective as a mosquito deterrent.[16] Betel nut chewing and cigarette smoking are enjoyable social behaviors for some people. Now with "no smoking" and "no junk food" campaigns in progress, I wonder if people will find an even unhealthier form of everyday entertainment.

One rather prosperous area in Mukah town was said in 2001 to be a hotbed of television-watching women who were obese, never exercised, and had diabetes and hypertension. Does this locus of a bad American lifestyle foretell the future of Sarawak?[17]

---

[10] Hose and MacDougall 1966, have a photograph of these statues (Plate 147).

[11] Ridu 1994.

[12] Sutlive and Sutlive 2001.

[13] Christensen 2002.

[14] Kedit 1982.

[15] Howden 1984.

[16] Baer 2004.

[17] Ironically, about 16% of pre-school children in Mukah District as a whole were undernourished in 2001, according to hospital records. One inland village, Kampung Teh, had a higher rate, 19% (E. Garit, personal communication).

Cooperative Methods

A third way also exists for health education and prevention of illness, between the conventional-modern and the traditional. Several examples of this third way, the cooperative way, exist for Sarawak. One example centered on a child nutrition program and a kindergarten for the Berawan.[18] Another was on coastal Malay villages in terms of preventing dengue.[19] A third was on coping with environmental health problems in an Iban longhouse.[20] All of these cases involved health education for the local population, but not in the conventional sense. Rather, local participation was essential for data gathering, problem solving, planning, actions, and obtaining results. This kind of work has improved the awareness of, and knowledge about, health problems in the three selected areas and empowered people to improve their living world. That is, instead of a community waiting for the government to intervene to address health-related problems, it now finds itself more in charge of its own destiny. This large accomplishment requires much time and effort both by community members and by the outside participants. As such, it can never be replicated in every village in Sarawak. But for those areas where it has been tried, it provides pay-offs not only in health improvement but also in self-esteem and local pride.

I once suggested another cooperative method to prevent or rectify health problems, one that is economical and not time-consuming for government workers, at least in the beginning. Dayak (or other) associations could sponsor essay contests open to secondary school students to write about their ideas for improving health in their local areas. Although the students who won prizes for their essays would not usually be regarded as sources of wisdom at home, with the prestige of the community association behind them—and the cooperation of local health professionals—their ideas might grow into improvements a whole village could be proud of.

A cross-over between traditional and modern methods of preventing illness involves modernists learning which remedies of traditional healers are efficacious and then using them.[21] For example, in East Kalimantan medical botanists interviewed Dayak healers about remedies by describing hypothetical cases of hepatitis, shingles, measles, ringworm, and other problems, often using pictures of the disease symptoms. Biomedical terms were not used. Instead, the healers were asked about the natural history and symptoms of the illness. Once an illness was recognized by a healer, she or he was asked how it was classified locally and its botanical

---

[18] Wong 1991.

[19] Crabtree et al. 2001. Dengue fever is centered in Southeast Asia; in 2001, there were an estimated 400,000 cases in the region. No treatment or cure exists for it.

[20] Andrews and Wong 2000.

[21] Leaman et al. 1995; Gollin 1997.

treatment. Relevant plants were collected for laboratory analysis later and for their commercial potential. Other villagers were asked what local remedies they used for common ailments such as headaches. Among other findings, herbal steam baths and face and body plasters were found to be popular in the area, although they are not fashionable in high-tech medical practice. Maybe the moderns are missing something. Likewise, given a low-calcium diet, pregnant Kayan women dosing themselves with powdered egg shells are benefitting their own and their offspring's nutrition, but this practice may not make it to a nutritionist's priority list.

Preventing AIDS is an entirely different challenge, as discussed in the next chapter.

CHAPTER EIGHT

HIV/AIDS AND OTHER SEXUALLY TRANSMITTED DISEASES (STDs)

A young Sarawak man gave me a conspiratorial wink as we passed by each other on a college walkway. We were both deviants—that is, we were unusual. I was an older woman in blue jeans and he was a cross-dresser with long tresses. Malaysia has quite a few cross-dressers—they're even traditional in some ritual situations. Some young ones work as prostitutes. Whenever I meet one I wonder if he has a STD such as AIDS, the acquired immune-deficiency syndrome. But, in fact, heterosexuals are the common victims of AIDS in Sarawak.[1]

STDs with the most serious health consequences include syphilis, gonorrhea, and the HIV viral infection that leads to AIDS. Already in the 1950s, United Nation workers in Sarawak observed a deputation of Iban women trekking to Kuching to urge the Medical Department to tackle the sterility then making inroads among them:

> Instead of...regarding their declining fertility as a visitation by the gods, the women recognized that the doctors could do something about it. And they probably can, because the epidemic of sterility is most likely due to the spread of venereal diseases...[2]

In the past, and continuing today, some Sarawak men work for months or years away from their families. The more they are away from home, the more likely they are to contract STDs. When, or if, the men return home, their wives are then vulnerable to STD transmission.

---

[1] Chong 1999.
[2] Calder 1954:48.

Sarawak has the highest rate of reported STDs in Malaysia. The state also has a low level of safe-sex practices.[3] In the year 2000 Sarawak had 2,500 *new* STD cases reported annually.[4] In 2001, about 40% of all reported STD cases in Sarawak were syphilis, 60% were gonorrhea, and less than 1% were AIDS. While STDs occur in all sectors of the Malaysian population, their significance is particularly acute in the commercial sex sector. No report seems to exist on the profile of women working in the sex sector in Sarawak, although one exists for West Malaysia.[5] If the situation in both places is similar, then some Sarawak prostitutes may think that a medical checkup, usually done at a private clinic, will prevent or cure AIDS. Some are probably single mothers. Some may have had an abortion. Some may insist their customers use condoms. Poorly educated girls and single women who lack skills for conventional work can earn far more as prostitutes than daytime workers earn. Many may be sending money home. With only fifty customers a month, a prostitute might net RM 3500.

AIDS

The world HIV epidemic started over 20 years ago. In biological terms the HIV virus causes AIDS, but AIDS is a growing epidemic in Southeast Asia largely for other reasons. Knowledge about AIDS and about safe-sex practices is woefully inadequate in Sarawak.[6] Beyond that, knowledge itself is of little use if attitudes are unrealistic about ways to prevent STDs.

There has been no mass screening for the HIV virus in Malaysia, only screening of those involved in high-risk activities, such as injecting drug users who may share hypodermic needles. Based on these studies, HIV/AIDS rates are rising in Malaysia as a whole, with 853 reported AIDS cases in 1990 versus 4,942 in 1992.[7] By 1998, 24,000 infections were known officially, mostly in men, but a better estimate is 60,000 infections.[8] By 2001 there were 40,049 known infections, with some 4,000 deaths.[9]

By the year 2000, Sarawak had 185 test-positive HIV carriers, with the majority of them estimated to be due to heterosexual contacts and most of them being in the 20 to 40 age group. By mid-2001, Sarawak had 309

---

[3] Rintos 2001; Chong 1999.

[4] *The Sunday Star*, 2 July, 2000, p. 12. The percentage of these cases in females was not stated.

[5] Shyamala Nagaraj and Siti Rohani Yahya 1998.

[6] Rabi'al and Kiyu 1995.

[7] Lye et al 1994.

[8] Rokiah Ismail 1998.

[9] Anonymous 2000a. Both Thailand and Cambodia have mounted successful "100% condom" campaigns, and Malaysia could benefit by following their example (Cohen 2001).

reported HIV carriers, of whom 40 had died of AIDS, suggesting that the number of infections increased 100% in about one year. By 2003, 20% of the victims were women, a much higher percentage than for Malaysia as a whole. By mid-2004 there were 424 HIV carriers in Sarawak.[10] The rate of new infections may now be accelerating in Sarawak, just as it is doing in Indonesia.[11]

AIDS is a reportable disease in Malaysia—along with gonococcal infections and syphilis—which occurs in prostitutes, their customers, and the customers' other sexual contacts. All the same, the Ministry of Health "has tended to keep its distance from the sex sector."[12] It seems to be a political hot potato. While prostitution is not illegal under criminal law in Malaysia, it is prohibited by Islamic law there.[13] As one expert wrote:

> An interesting question is whether religion actually has any significant influence in reducing either the supply of, or demand for, prostitutes. The answer would appear to be no, although all the major religions condemn prostitution and extramarital relations.[14]

In general, prostitution seems to be immune to being either criminalized or decriminalized, to being either prohibited or regulated. It is often conveniently ignored. If it is embedded in Malaysia, its health effects cannot be ignored for long. The most obvious effects are in the spread of sexually transmitted diseases, particularly AIDS.

I tried to estimate the impact of the AIDS epidemic on Sarawak by taking some data from a 1998 paper on West Malaysia and applying it across "the pond."[15] First I did the arithmetic using a Sarawak population of 2.1 million in the year 2000 multiplied by the published estimate that 0.237% of the population were prostitutes. This equaled 4,980 of them. Then I did the arithmetic in a second way suggested by the 1998 paper, assuming that most prostitutes were in the urban areas and that half of Sarawakians (a million) lived in them. I rounded off the total number of prostitutes to 5,000, a number smaller than that reported for the city of Kuala Lumpur alone. This implies that about 0.5% of Sarawak's urban

---

[10] *Bernama*, 29 July, 2004.

[11] Cohen 2005.

[12] Lin 1998:96.

[13] Soliciting, pimping, and trafficking in women or girls are illegal, I'm told, but I don't know if working in a brothel is considered soliciting.

[14] Lin 1998:14.

[15] Shyamala Nagaraj and Siti Rohani Yahya 1998.

residents are prostitutes.[16] If each prostitute averages only 100 *different* "clients" per year, this yields a maximum of 500,000 possible client HIV infections per year in Sarawak. That number may be nearly all the men in the state. And they could infect 500,000 wives at home.

Unrealistic? Of course. Unlike South Africa, Sarawak is still in the early stages of the AIDS epidemic.[17] Perhaps few Sarawak men have sex with prostitutes. No one knows how many prostitutes there are in Sarawak or how many of them are HIV-infected.[18] Moreover, condom usage might become fashionable, as may marital fidelity, even celibacy. But the potential for a large epidemic is present, nonetheless.

Major HIV epidemics tend to occur in areas where unprotected sex is common in heterosexual contacts.[19] Most HIV infections in Sarawak are due to heterosexual transmission, rather than bi- or homo-sexual transmission, or to any association with drug addiction. This means that women in Sarawak are more vulnerable to HIV infections than those in West Malaysia.[20] Unfortunately, the research literature is largely silent about HIV/AIDS in Sarawak women. In a relevant study in Kelantan, 171 women were tested for HIV and syphilis at the only drug-rehabilitation center for women in Malaysia.[21] Some of the women had acquired HIV by sharing needles during drug usage, but 48% of them had been sex workers. Moreover, 60% of these women said their sexual partners never used condoms. This is significant because condoms are readily available in Malaysia (which, in fact, manufactures them) and they do protect against HIV transmission.[22] Since HIV is more often transmitted to women sex workers by male clients than the other way around, it comes as no surprise that 14% of the 171 women were found to be HIV-positive. Even more of the women tested positive for syphilis, 39%. However, sex work was not correlated with the presence of HIV in this Kelantan study, although sharing drug needles was. This would not be the expectation for Sarawak.

---

[16] In 1984 more than 700 Iban women prostitutes were registered at a government clinic in Sibu for required health check-ups; about 4% of the sample interviewed had been diagnosed as having a STD (Sutlive 1991).

[17] See: http://www.census/gov/ipc/hiv/malaysia.pdf.

[18] One report I've seen said that 892 foreigners *suspected* of being sex workers were arrested in Sarawak between 1989 and mid-1992. Filipinos were the largest subgroup (553). Foreign prostitutes are "prohibited immigrants" subject to deportation when arrested for vice (Shyamala Nagaraj and Siti Rohani Yahya 1998). These authors also report that among 44 prostitutes they interviewed who were working in West Malaysia, one was Iban and one was Kadazan.

[19] Jha et al. 2001.

[20] I do not know if health workers require HIV carriers to notify their sexual partners or if Malaysia, or Sarawak, requires partner notification for any STD.

[21] Wai et al. 1996.

[22] It seems that single men or women buying condoms in a Sarawak pharmacy risk social censure because sexuality is only condoned in marriage by government policy.

In Sarawak prostitution is all too common and glue sniffing rather than intravenously injecting opiates is the usual drug behavior. Sarawak probably benefits by being away from the supply of drugs on the Asian mainland; also, glue is cheaper than heroin. For Sarawak women, then, one would expect HIV to be correlated with sex work and, increasingly, for HIV infection to become common in wives whose husbands were customers of sex workers or were generally promiscuous. Already in Sarawak, couples made up 30% of the HIV cases by the late 1990s.[23] This home-based transmission clearly victimizes women.[24]

While condom usage helps greatly to prevent the spread of the AIDS virus, information on condoms is ambiguous. In a small study of West Malaysian prostitutes, over 60% of them said they made their customers use condoms. And certainly condoms are available in many pharmacies and other venues. But grassroots usage may be lax at best. At least in one area Iban women considered condoms to be "funny."[25] Moreover, I was advised not to mention condoms as a means of preventing AIDS in any village, as this subject might offend the residents. Male circumcision can also reduce the chance of an HIV infection, but it is unknown if circumcision reduces an HIV-infected man's ability to transmit the virus.[26]

Malaysian women's groups have given some attention to the danger of sexually transmitted diseases for prostitutes. A campaign that included concern for prostitutes' health was mounted by the umbrella group NCWO (National Council of Women's Organizations) in the 1990s. Non-governmental organizations have also urged the federal government to fund safe-sex education in schools.[27] The government so far declines.

Another group suggested as a potential factor in the spread of HIV is fishermen who sail between Southeast Asian ports. I have seen no study of this group for Sarawak, but in Malaysia as a whole fishermen are over-represented among AIDS victims.[28] Likewise, "invisible" but sexually-

---

[23] Chong 1999.

[24] Sutlive (1991) reported the expectation that Iban husbands would philander when working afield, it being one reason they took to traveling (see also Huang 2002). Grijpstra (1976) noted that when husbands are away form home, they often behave like bachelors. Catterall (1981) reported that doctors seldom ask men treated for STDs about their sexual contacts; this is a disservice to women who may thus have become infected. While Linklater (1990) held that both Iban husbands and wives were sometimes promiscuous whenever they were not living together, Kedit (1991) held that Iban moral values of marital fidelity and clean living kept most men away from brothels when they worked in the towns.

[25] Edwards 1999. Also, Bario men shun condoms (J. M. Lensy, personal communication). While some Iban prostitutes in Sibu ask men to use condoms, the men often refuse (Sutlive 1991). Men's complaints about condoms are rebutted on p. 193 in Burns et al. 1997.

[26] Cohen 2005. Iban once practiced circumcision on older boys after numbing them by immersion in water (Sutlive and Sutlive 2001).

[27] Anonymous 2002.

[28] Huang 2000.

active teenagers who drop out of school and migrate to urban areas for unskilled jobs have received little attention in Sarawak.

Throughout the world women are vulnerable to HIV infection because of poverty, poor education, violence, and cultural norms.[29] If a woman already has another STD, that can make her physiologically even more vulnerable. Because pregnant women who are HIV-positive can pass on the virus to their offspring, these women are tested for HIV in Sarawak. If positive, both they and their newborns are treated. So far, Sarawak has seen little of this problem, nor has it seen a high rate of HIV-positives in sex workers. Its HIV pool is in the general population. While about 2% of people with other STDs were found to have HIV in Sarawak in 1994, less than 1% of them had HIV a year later.[30]

The General Hospital in Kuching has a treatment program for HIV-infected people that plays a large role in monitoring and aiding them. Patients there can receive the full 3-dose medication for ameliorating the infection. Patients come into this program because it is the most comprehensive in the state and also because, if they live elsewhere, they can be away from the eyes of their fellow residents. In Kuching they are not in the embarrassing position of having to tell their family about their infection. This points up one reason why HIV is more a social than a biological problem.

Another social component of AIDS is children whose mothers or both parents have died of AIDS. These orphans number in the thousands in Malaysia as a whole and are a small but growing problem in Sarawak. Some are from poor families in which grandmothers or other close kin do not have the funds or extra time for raising them. So far, this aspect of the AIDS epidemic has received little attention.

Health workers have publicized the threat of AIDS to some extent in Sarawak. In Lundu District, nurses have given talks to village women about AIDS, pointing out that the women needed to be aware of AIDS to safeguard their own health. The women rejoined that the talks should be given to the men, as they are the ones who bring it in from outside. The women "just stay at home," they said.[31] These women realize they can be put at risk, not because of their own sexual behavior but their partner's behavior. While the nurses hoped the women would discuss STDs with

---

[29] Quinn and Overbaugh 2005.

[30] See: http://www.census/gov/ipc/hiv/malaysia.pdf.

[31] However, in the 1970s Grijpstra (1976:10) mentioned "girls who earn an income soliciting members of the armed forces... Women engaged in the oldest profession are by no means treated as outcasts." More recently, some young Bidayuh women worked in brothels and traveling prostitutes visited Bidayuh areas near Bau on weekends (Kiyu 1993). In like vein, promiscuity in men is not unknown. One can only wonder about the village man considered to be the local champion in adultery (Grijpstra 1976).

their husbands, they decided also to give these talks to the men at a later date.

Health education about STDs in Sarawak could benefit by targeting the most vulnerable parts of the population. A well-designed study in northern Thailand found that HIV was much more common in some ethnic groups than in others, in younger women but older men, in male patrons of sex workers, in women who worked in the sex sector, in people who had some pre-existing STD, and in those from very poor areas. A comparable study would be useful in Sarawak. If the Thai results apply to the Sarawak situation, STD education could well be targeted to poor people (whether urban squatters or villagers), young women who are school-dropouts working away from home, patients with other STDs, and commercial sex workers and their customers.

Viruses like HIV are not the pawns of cultural beliefs, so cultural beliefs must change if the HIV problem is to be overcome. Prompt action can fend off this self-inflicted and widespread pain and its long-term economic costs. But just as it would be difficult to cure Malaysians of eating polished rice (while discarding the nutritious bran), it may be even harder to extirpate an entrenched commercial sex trade and make condoms readily acceptable.

> HIV and Culture
>
> Malaysia has long been "in denial" about AIDS.[32] To ignore reality, deviants are blamed for the spread of AIDS. Deviants are defined as drug users, foreigners, and prostitutes, among others. The claim that giving sex education in schools or promoting general condom use is contrary to a country's culture often reflects the view of urban elites. They see HIV-infected people as deviants from the correct way of living, proving ipso facto that the elite worldview is morally superior. Authorities hew to this line to maintain their political power. The media in Southeast Asian countries does not dispute the authorities' view because it is insecure and often lacks objective information. The media, especially the non-English media, may also regard drug users and sex workers—usually poor people—as unimportant, on top of being deviant. NGOs, public health workers, and others who deal with these cultural constraints face a challenging road ahead.

Gonorrhea

Gonorrhea was evidently common in Sarawak in the past. The people of the Upper Tinjar, largely Kenyah, were said to be dying out in the 1950s due to the high incidence of gonorrhea there.[33] It may also have

---

[32] Wolffers 1997.
[33] De Zulueta 1957.

contributed to the high sterility attributed to Iban women in the 1950s. However, among the Iban and Berawan, induced abortions were once used to stop pre-marital pregnancies as they evoked social censure and shame.[34] In both groups, much sterility was thought to be due to induced abortions.

Gonorrhea is a disease for which there is no vaccine and no long-term cure for sexually active people. Once infected, people can transmit the disease for several months. After this period, they become susceptible to re-infection. For this reason the disease can persist even in small, scattered populations in Sarawak. Although it might seem a paradox, gonorrhea impacts women's health, even though many infected women have no direct symptoms. Men are more likely to have symptoms, and when they do, they can readily obtain antibiotic treatment that clears the infection. But for women, gonorrhea can produce pelvic inflammatory disease, which is a leading cause of sterility and associated ectopic pregnancy. If this is a problem in Sarawak, it has not been well studied, despite past concerns about sterility in some cultural groups.

Syphilis

When A. W. Nieuwenhuis visited the Kayan of the Upper Mahakam in Dutch Borneo in the 1890s, he found syphilis in every family and assumed it was hereditary there.[35] It was later shown to be a bacterial disease. I have seen no research report on syphilis in Sarawak. One reason may be that, although syphilis is fairly common in the state, it is treatable. As is the case for HIV, pregnant women are tested for syphilis and, if necessary, they and their newborns are treated for it.

---

[34] See Padoch (1982) on the Iban; Metcalf (1974) on the Berawan.

[35] Nieuwenhuis 1929.

CHAPTER NINE

MENTAL HEALTH

Mental illness has strong cultural dimensions among the Melanau. A common mental disorder among postpartum Melanau women in the Mukah area is called *meruyan*. Melanau do not regard it as a psychosis or as being identical to postpartum depression. It is usually attributed to eating tabooed foods such as a strong-smelling fruit or fish. Health centers and traditional healers both treat *meruyan*.[1]

Despite the tendency of "scientific" medicine to denigrate traditional health beliefs and practices, some astute medical workers are well aware of their efficacy. They understand the benefits of shamans, *pawang*, *manang*, *dukun*, *bomoh*s, and the like. As one doctor put it:

> Bomohs and so on are very good with mental illness. They often treat the whole family, the father, mother and all the others. And they treat the patient in ways familiar to his conception of things.[2]

Interestingly, genealogies of Iban *manang* (traditional healers) collected by Robert Barrett, a psychiatrist, show a trend toward paramedical staff positions in the health field in recent years. The Iban see this as healing power descending through time in *manang* families.[3]

While Southeast Asian cultures are noted for their concern to keep human psyches in harmony, forms of mental disturbance have long been recognized in Sarawak. The Bidayuh distinguished dull-idiotic behavior from insanity, which includes mania and paranoid schizophrenia, but

---

[1] Appleton 2004.
[2] Wiebe and Rahim Said 1980:183.
[3] Barrett 1993.

epilepsy was not considered a mental illness.[4] Likewise, a bad temperament that did not interfere with the ability to function in the farming society was considered to be within the range of permissible behavior. Some mental illnesses among the Bidayuh were said to be caused by heredity, others by grief, bad air entering the head, evil spirits of the dead, or other factors. If people transgressed social rules, the spirits might retaliate by making them insane. Traditional treatment of mental illness, for both Bidayuh and Iban, involves a *manang* performing certain rituals. Mental retardation, however, is not considered treatable.

Iban traditionally viewed most illness as due to supernatural beings, including mental illness. Violating a taboo commonly caused mental problems, including epilepsy and violent behavior. Social disgrace or economic failure could also precipitate mental illness, as could anemia and a few other physical factors in the Iban view.[5] Iban recognized the categories of chronic mania, autism, epilepsy, senile dementia, running amok, mental retardation, and other types of mental dysfunction. Longhouse people largely tolerated deviant behavior as long as it did not endanger the community.

Malays were long known for running amok and for *latah*, but also in the 1960s for neurosyphilis, according to the records of the Sarawak Mental Hospital in Kuching.[6] *Latah* is a condition involving socially inappropriate echolalia, plus imitative gestures or movements. In Sarawak it seems to be restricted to women and it is not regarded as an illness. It may be a means of self-expression for those having difficulty coping with life's stresses, but may involve a hypersensitivity to startling.[7] It has been found among the Iban and Bidayuh of Lundu, Saribas Iban, and Muslim Melanau, but not among non-Muslim Melanau.[8] It is lowland-coastal in distribution, not being found in the interior of Sarawak.

To alleviate severe depression, Melanau once went through several stages of treatment, starting with herbal medicine and charms. This was followed by anointing a sago-pith spirit image and also the patient, plus other rituals. Then government or Chinese medicine was tried. Finally, a *payun* ceremony was held that could last for nine nights. It involved drumming, incense, and trance.[9]

Despite traditional views that spirits can cause disease, especially mental illness, some modern Sarawakians say, "We have no *antus* (spirits) here." Yet, in their parents or grandparents time the world was full of unseen but real spirits—good, bad, or capricious. This enabled traditional

---

[4] Nissan and Schmidt 1967.

[5] Schmidt 1996. Iban have 42 terms for mental problems (Sutlive and Sutlive 2001).

[6] Schmidt 1996.

[7] Simons 1992.

[8] Winzeler 1995.

[9] Barnes 1966.

healers to treat conceptual, or mental, problems in a holistic fashion.[10] Indeed, not only the patient but the whole village reccived revitalization. That sense of local solidarity was considered the basis of everyone's health. Even today, a local group may eschew modern medicine despite imminent danger to the patient. Harris told how an Iban woman dying of dengue fever was given community attention and therapy rather than an ambulance ride to hospital that might have saved her life.[11] That community solidarity was valued as an indication of the superiority of local knowledge over alien ideas. The mental health of the community was thereby preserved.

Traditional farming practices in Sarawak supported mental health: rice was not only produced and eaten, it sustained religious and other social activities. In contrast today, cash cropping for oil palm, pepper, or cocoa production provides neither food security nor does it have religious or social significance in Sarawak cultures.

Sarawak had, in the 1990s, very few psychiatrists or psychiatric social workers. For psychiatric patients living at home, rather than in an institution, community psychiatric nurses provide help in coping with life, including educating the patient's family about the problem at hand. Treatment of psychiatric out-patients and in-patients of the Sarawak Mental Hospital in Kuching has recently been studied.[12] The out-patients spanned five cultural groups in (Malay, Chinese, Bidayuh, Iban, and Kayan), many of them living in poverty-stricken families. Most of the patients were diagnosed as having schizophrenic psychosis but a few had a "learning disability" or epilepsy. While the health professionals tried to explain the patient's problem in biomedical terms, this study showed that the patient's family often regarded the abnormality as being supernaturally caused, an explanation acceptable in the local culture. In addition, this explanation put no blame on the patient for his or her problem. Other explanations commonly proffered by families for the abnormality included work or marriage stresses, or prior fevers that caused a vulnerability to illness. Most of the families had tried psychotherapy from traditional healers before seeking psychiatric treatment for their family member. Psychiatric conditions were more likely to be tolerated in male family members than in females. Women could be forbidden to have social outings on their own, for example, while men tended to go out to socialize with their friends. In some cases women who were considered "immodest" were actually confined at home, but male patients did not get

---

[10] However, some Iban, for example, have long been skeptical about shamanistic practices (Barrett 1993). This group includes people who have received some modern schooling but also older Iban, even some *manang* themselves. But even when the practices are suspect, the effectiveness of shamanistic treatment is more widely acknowledged.

[11] Harris 2001.

[12] Crabtree 1999, 2003, 2005.

similarly labeled in terms of sexually-suggestive behavior. Two problems faced by many of these families with a psychiatric patient at home were, one, the cost of maintaining someone who could not obtain a job and, two, avoiding conflict with, or censure from, neighbors and the community. Families often isolated themselves from their social world.

In-patient women were seemingly unpaid laborers at the mental hospital, perhaps as a form of occupational therapy, and in general were disadvantaged more than male patients there. The attitudes of hospital professionals toward patients were negative, in line with the stigma attached to mental problems locally.

A clinical case study has been published on a schizophrenic Iban woman living in a longhouse with her adoptive mother (her maternal aunt who was barren).[13] In this case, as for some of the out-patients studied in Kuching, the patient saw spirits. When her problem was recognized, she was first taken to private doctors and later to the Kuching General Hospital, which transferred her to the Sarawak Mental Hospital. She was then 25 years old. She was later in and out of a district psychiatric unit. She received medication at these government facilities and later as an out-patient through her local clinic, but her hallucinations, delusions, and depression persisted. She was also treated by three Iban healers and by a Christian healing ceremony. None of them were successful. Many serious family troubles preceded the patient's diagnosis of schizophrenia.[14] This Iban patient wanted to get married and to leave her adoptive mother's tight control over her life. The Iban, however, regard schizophrenia as incurable and censure it. Even siblings of such a patient may be stigmatized as being unsuitable for marriage, one fear being that children may inherit schizophrenia.[15] However, the patient had several advantages over similar patients living in urban areas. Her longhouse provided a focal center to her life and she had many farming and domestic duties, which she did very well. At the same time, she was forbidden much "outside" socializing, such as occurs at Iban festivals and funerals.

A survey of medical records recently led to an estimate of schizophrenia occurring in the range of 0.4% to 1.1% in a Sarawak Iban population located in one river catchment area.[16] Most of these patients were characterized by insomnia and aggression prior to their diagnosis.

Forced relocation in Sarawak may also contribute to mental problems. Anecdotal evidence comes from the Bakun dam hydro-refugees. The men

---

[13] Barrett 1997.

[14] In the United States today, this might familiarly be described as a kind of post-traumatic stress disorder.

[15] According to the *Adat Iban 1993*, one recognized cause for divorce is if a spouse has been mentally ill or leprous for two years or longer, with certification by a hospital (Sutlive and Sutlive 2001).

[16] Barrett et al. 2005.

took to drinking too much; even some women did. This has been described as due to a social separation syndrome, in which people feel devalued, conflicts occur over roles and aspirations, and people grieve over the loss of social integrity. People are disoriented, with consequences to their health.[17]

Sarawakians know that mental illness is not easily curable. While they gravitate to health clinics for illnesses that can be cured, there is an understandable ambivalence about how to cope with other illnesses. Many prefer the comfort of traditional approaches. Better the devil you know...

On a global scale, there is evidence that men and women experience mental problems somewhat differently. After the tsunami of 2004, relief money was handed out in Tamil Nadu. Many of the men spent it on drinking, but money given to women was spent much more wisely. The women dealt with the tsunami aftermath not by drinking but by depression and anxiety.[18] Throughout the world, it seems that women are more prone to depression, anxiety, and phobias than men.[19] While men tend to externalize their problems, women internalize them. This may be related to difference in sex hormones between men and women. Primate studies, for instance, have shown that testosterone is related to aggression. But learned responses are also important for men's and women's maladaptive behaviors, whether anti-social (men) or depression (women).

In the case of the Bakun hydro-refugees, their mental upsets are likely the result of their everyday concerns and not primarily a health problem.[20] By analogy with the tsunami disaster victims, their basic needs are reestablishing their community cohesion, having enough money to send their children to school, and living in a healthy, natural environment. That is, they don't need psychiatric help, they need the bare amenities of a normal life.

---

[17] Appell 1980.
[18] Miller 2005b.
[19] Holden 2005.
[20] Miller 2005a.

CHAPTER TEN

LIFE, DEATH, AND DEMOGRAPHY

The Dutch historian, Han Knapen, proposed that the Borneo rainforest was once intact because populations were sparse. Population growth was kept low mainly by the interplay of disease and environment.[1] The main cause of illness and childhood death was malaria, at least in the interior, followed by intestinal diseases (dysentery and cholera) and smallpox. Cholera and smallpox epidemics swept through the land as outsiders infiltrated it. That is, forest sustainability was lost not because of colonialism or its aftermath *per se* but simply by newcomers increasingly ravaging the landscape and introducing their infectious diseases.[2] Today, both the environment and the health issues in Borneo's Sarawak are quite different from several centuries ago.

The basic geography of Sarawak is tripartite, a coastal plain, the hills, and the highland interior. The plain takes up half the land and holds over 90% of the population. The hills and highlands cover the other half but have less than 10% of the population. This distribution skews the availability of health services toward the lowlands. It also has implications for environmental factors that affect people's health. For example, population density on the plain alters coastal ecosystems, making them more vulnerable to health hazards such as water-borne diseases, especially during flooding.

Demography intersects with health in sometimes surprising ways. Immigrants who bring diseases into the state, or coastal people who travel upriver to trade with immunologically vulnerable people in the interior, are unsurprising examples. In contrast, Bernard Sellato noted that Dayaks of the Apo Kayan plateau of Kalimantan in the 1960s took action when Dutch imports of salt waned. The Dayaks stepped up trading for home-

---

[1] Other factors may have been birth control (via infanticide, abortifacients, or mechanical abortion), prolonged lactation, high female workload, warfare, or human sacrifice.

[2] Knapen 1998.

made salt from Sarawak and many emigrated, some to Sarawak. Perhaps this was simply due to a salt craving, but what the migrants gained was iodine (in the Sarawak salt) sufficient to forestall serious goiter problems. For those who stayed behind in Kalimantan, goiter became a common sight.[3] What Sarawak gained was more people.

An interesting conjecture is that headhunting, while it did not kill many people or cause societal collapse as smallpox did, kept many Dayak societies closely-knit and geographically isolated, almost as if they were in quarantine. With the crack-down on headhunting in Sarawak during the Brooke era and later, this health advantage evaporated as social and economic exchanges among groups increased.[4]

A corollary of headhunting, such as in the Iban case, was enemy capture. A captive became a family slave and could be adopted into it. Captives could directly expand the Iban population and workforce while dead heads could not. This in-migration might also have exposed the capturing group to alien diseases, but little is know about this aspect of history.

Another intersection of demography and health issues involves the density of the population. Some infectious diseases cannot persist in small, scattered populations because the population either dies off or becomes immune. This was long the case for smallpox. Those in a small group who survived a smallpox epidemic became permanently immune to the virus and so the disease disappeared locally. The virus then had to be re-introduced from the outside at the right time, usually when the next generation of susceptible victims came into existence.

Also, while growing hill rice does not usually provide enough calories to sustain a large population, growing wet rice can foster population increase. A downside is that flooded rice paddies can support many breeding mosquitoes whereas hill swiddens minimize this problem.

High population density has many health correlates. Urbanization invariably means crowding, and thus diseases such as dengue have become associated with urban areas. People have standing water around their houses, whether in rain-filled discarded containers or intentionally left in flower pots. The mosquito larvae of Aedes aegypti, a vector of dengue, thrive in these novel environments. Also, if urban water supplies are not kept to a high standard, cholera can become widespread. This is of particular concern in squatter settlements around cities. Crowded resettlement areas, such as those resulting from the Bakun dam project, also have "urban" health problems. Temporary housing quarters for workers at any large development site are of similar concern.

Sedentization of mobile forest groups over the past two generations likewise led to a change, from a low to a high malaria situation. In 1971

---

[3] Sellato 1993.

[4] Knapen 1998.

some Penan were still resisting moving downstream because they thought there was more disease there, an opinion that health workers didn't dispute. After the Punan Busang were sedentized, their population went from 150 to 75 in three years. Moreover, 20% of the oldest generation had no surviving offspring in 1971, partly due to sterility and partly to a very high infant mortality rate—over 25%.[5]

As for the general demography of both urban and rural areas, modern times have generally lowered family size. In the Limbang watershed living conditions have declined for swidden farmers because of large-scale logging by others plus government restrictions on using the people's own lands for farming and forest resources.[6] The deforestation and resulting erosion in the area has produced poor river quality and poor soil fertility. The lives (and health) of farming people have also been affected in other ways. Since most children now go to primary school, they do not help much in farm work or daytime babysitting. While this makes farming harder for women, a counter trend has been that family sizes have been getting smaller. On the one hand, there are now fewer mouths to feed so subsistence farming is less pressured. On the other hand, schooling adds extra costs to households. To survive a variety of modern challenges, a majority of the women in one study said that they used contraceptives to limit family size.[7] To them, educating a few children to cope with pell-mell modernity is better than having many children to help in traditional work.[8]

Basic demographic data can produce estimates of crude birth rates (CBRs) and crude death rates (CDRs). They are the number of people born and the number that die annually per 1,000 population, respectively. These rates plus migration rates determine changes in population size and structure through time.

Many factors affect the birth rate. They include biological ones such as sterility and social ones such as age at marriage, induced abortions, contraception, and the extent of divorce and widowhood.[9] In the past, the age for a first marriage was about 15 years for both sexes in groups such as the Iban, putting girls at risk of pregnancy at an early age. Family planning clinics established in the 1960s in major towns became an important factor in lowering the birth rate in Sarawak.

---

5 Oldrey 1972; Ellis 1972.

6 Heyser 1995.

7 By 1970 Iban women were reported to be the largest cultural group to attend the family planning clinic in Sibu (Sutlive 1978).

8 Joekes 1994.

9 Berawan women used herbal medicine to abort a pre-marital pregnancy, in order to avoid shame (Metcalf 1974).

The birth rate and infant death rate were once widely viewed as an index of overall health conditions.[10] These data are still useful today to assess health trends, but they are not the only ones. To get a better grasp on reality, it is important to know maternal death rates, sex ratios by age group, age at first marriage, morbidity rates, and other data that contribute to the real-life health picture.

For example, a generation ago Rejang Iban had many children in the under-10 age bracket, amounting to 37% of the population.[11] In the 1990s, Rejang Iban were reported to have only 20% in this bracket.[12] Batang Ai had 25% in this bracket.[13] Lundu had fewer yet, 20%.[14] Taking these reports on population structure together, we can see that large local differences have existed in space and time. The differences will be due to some mixture of age-specific birth rates, death rates, and in- versus out-migration rates.

Sex ratio data offer clues to the survival success of the two sexes. The ratio varies among areas and cultural groups. For the Iban, the male:female ratio in Lundu was 0.94, in Batang Ai 0.93, in the Rejang area 0.80, and in Song-Kanowit 0.79 in 1980.[15] The male deficit was typically in the 20–49 age range, suggesting that many men were not only absent from their villages but were outside of Sarawak, perhaps in Brunei or Sabah.[16] By themselves, sex ratios less than 1.0 imply that women survive better than men, as seems to be the case in rich countries. But when men have left home, state, and even country (one Sarawakian took a job in Mexico), these ratios can be misleading in terms of understanding women's health. If women do survive less well than men in Sarawak, several questions arise. Indeed, the official sex ratio for Sarawak overall for 1990 shows more males than females (1.03), despite having male deficits in the 25–34 age range undoubtedly associated with men working in distant venues.[17]

One survey of rural Iban and Malay women in Miri District shows some of the demographic factors in rural health a generation ago.[18] At that time the women studied had averaged four to five pregnancies, even though they ranged in age from 18 to 49 years. This implies that completed fertility for these women would be greater than five

---

[10] In 1986 the CBR for Sarawak was 109 per 1,000 population; the infant mortality rate was not available, due to omissions in reporting (*Demographic Yearbook* 1994).

[11] Ogihara et al. 1972a.

[12] Strickland and Ulijaszek 1994.

[13] Kedit 1993.

[14] Winzeler 1995.

[15] Baer et al. 2001.

[16] Padoch (1982) found that 23 of the 24 Engkari men on *bejalai* (traveling) in the 1970s were outside of Sarawak, most of them being in timber camps in Sabah.

[17] *Demographic Yearbook* 1994.

[18] Goto et al. 1974.

pregnancies when they reached menopause, assuming that all of them would survive to that stage in life.[19] The women in the study reported having about 3% of their pregnancies end in miscarriage, abortion, or stillbirth, although they may have forgotten to count all of these calamities in their past. More than 90% of their pregnancies ended up in home births. Among the home births, 1% had no help at all in delivery while traditional midwives or family members helped the rest. Half of the infants born were breastfed, 12% were fed condensed or powdered milk, and the rest were fed by both means. For the 430 live births recorded in this survey, the infant death rate was 7.5% and the death rate for children 1 to 9 years of age was 4.1%, with more Iban infants dying than Malay infants (8.4% versus 5.1%). At that time (1972), the official infant mortality rate for Sarawak was about 3.1%, given that there were 31,281 registered live births and 966 registered infant deaths in that year.[20] However, under-registration was then known to be widespread. In the 1972 Iban-Malay survey, fever, diarrhea, and vomiting were said to precede infant deaths. The survey area at that time did not have a health clinic or potable water supplies for villages, and there was much poverty. However, since the 1970s much has changed for the better. Between 1972 and 1986, for example, the infant death rate had declined from 3.1% to 1% in Sarawak.[21]

Recent Census Information[22]

According to government records, the Sarawak population was growing at a rate of 2.2% per year in 1991–1995. In the year 2000 Sarawak's population was over 2 million, with some 48,000 live births and almost 9,000 recorded deaths, giving a natural increase of 39,000 per year, assuming in- and out-migration rates are equal. This means that the population is still growing at a fast rate, about 2% per year. If this trend continues, the population will double over the next 30 years. The three main reasons for this demographic success are increases in scientific discoveries in many fields, increases in reliable health information, and increases in the availability of health services.

The Sarawak population is still quite young on the whole, with over 30% being under the age of 15 years. While longevity is inching up, few people are old, that is, over the cut-off age of 59. In contrast, the erstwhile Sarawak visitor, Alfred Wallace, lived to be 90 years of age, a fact that would astound most Sarawakians even today.

---

[19] The completed (total) fertility rate for women in Malaysia was 3.2 in 2002, twice the rate in Singapore (http://www.prb.org/).

[20] *Annual Statistical Bulletin* 1978.

[21] Sarawak Medical and Health Services 1986.

[22] Information in this section is largely based on *Yearbook of Statistics, Sarawak* 2003.

While Iban make up 29% of the population and are the largest cultural group, their live birth rate is the lowest, while their death rate is in the intermediate range.[23] As such, their natural rate of population increase is much lower than for other Sarawakians, such as the Chinese, Malays, and other indigenous groups. These "other indigenous groups," in fact, have the highest recorded rates of population increase.

The low rate of increase in the Iban may be the result of several factors, but one possibility can be dismissed: their infant death rate is much lower than that of other groups. Notably, it is about half that of Bidayuh, who have the highest recorded rate of infant deaths. However, Bidayuh seem to survive better after the infant stage, since they have a lower over-all death rate than the Iban do. The reasons for this variability are obscure.

Population data on deaths are as basic as those on births. Worldwide, deaths in infancy are higher than for other age groups, except for people at the end of the human lifespan. The infant mortality rate per 1,000 live births (IMR) was estimated to be 61 in 1970 and 34 in 1980 for all Sarawak indigenous groups.[24] In the 1960–1970 decade, unlike recently, the rate in Iban was about 150, or 15%, much higher than for other groups. This produced a low life expectancy for Iban, about 44 years at that time.[25]

What do people die of in Sarawak now? Of the 9,000 deaths in the state in 2000, perhaps less than half were medically certified. This guess is based on the fact that for 1999 only about 3,150 deaths were certified. (I have not seen comparable data for 2000.) Based on the figures for 1999, we can get some idea of common causes of death in the state. The highest recorded cause was diseases of the circulatory system, accounting for over 10% of total deaths, mainly due to heart malfunction. Cancer was the second highest recorded cause, with cancers affecting most parts of the body. Accidents took third place, mainly involving motor vehicles. In fourth place was infections disease; here, septicemia was the most common culprit.[26] If we ignore the uncertified deaths, we might interpret these findings as showing that Sarawak is moving from a past age of vulnerability to infectious diseases, especially in childhood, toward a future of "developed" diseases that occur mainly in adults. People are now living longer, but all of us still have to die somehow.

---

[23] Sterility can lower the birth rate. In 1970, 20% of Iban women 40–44 years of age were still childless, indicating female (or male) sterility (Lam 1983). Sterility can result from STDs, perhaps brought home by men. Sutlive (1991) noted that husbands philander on *bejalai*, it being one reason for men to undertake traveling. However, the birth rate may also go down as a result of *bejalai*, if men are away for years. A few never return, it is said.

[24] Leete and Kwok 1986. For all of Malaysia, the IMR was 11 in 1996, according to United Nations data. For Sarawak as a whole, it was 7 in 1996.

[25] Lam 1983.

[26] The maternal mortality rate hovered around 0.4 per 1,000 live births in 1990–1997 (http://sarawak.health.gov.my/). By 1999 it was down to 0.2 per 1000.

For people living far from health centers, however, infectious diseases can still be a terror. In early 2005, 13 children and one adult Penan died in Sarawak during a measles epidemic that struck 66 people in the longhouse at Sungai Urun. These Penan had never been exposed to measles before. The outbreak occurred after a man and wife returned to the longhouse from elsewhere, possibly bringing the virus with them.[27] Accidents in remote areas also occur regularly. For example, Sarawak had 34 logging-related deaths in 1999 and was on its way to a higher number in 2000.[28]

Unanswered Questions

To obtain a fuller picture of demographics in Sarawak, more research is needed than has been the case so far. A fuller picture is important because demographic data illuminate not only research in allied disciplines but practical considerations for governmental agencies, including health departments.

Researchers who can benefit from demographic data include anthropologists, sociologists, medical historians, human geneticists, and ecologists, among others.[29] Research questions that bear on demography include the role of endemic and epidemic disease in population groups, genetic factors important for survival, and the biosocial adaptations that contribute to a group's long-term prospects. Much basic work in demography remains to be done to give coherence to studies in the biological and social sciences, and the humanities, in Sarawak.

One research area that combines demographic and health questions is the history of the Iban expansion from Kalimantan into northern Borneo. While Iban are the largest Sarawak group today and the most widespread geographically, this was not always so. A number of fascinating questions arise about this expansion. Was it a slow, steadily expanding "front" of dispersers, or did groups "leapfrog" right and left across space? Were the pioneers individual adventurers or whole kin groups? Was the expansion based primarily on Iban ability in warfare (pulling them outward) or on farming success leading to overpopulation (pushing them outward)? Or did drought years or epidemics provide the push? While such questions envision only sharp contrasts, reality may lie somewhere in the zone between these extremes. These in-between possibilities compound the difficulties in trying to envision plausible scenarios for the expansion. We are, at the moment, forced to fall back on impressions. Based on what little is known about Iban demography over the past few centuries, the salient features of the Iban expansion seem to be (1) generally high birth rates, (2) high childhood death rates, (3) short lifespans, perhaps especially for

---

[27] Anonymous 2005.

[28] *Sarawak Tribune*, 25 July, 2000, p. 8.

[29] See Appell (1969) on the importance of census work in anthropology.

multiparous women, (4) a preference for village or areal endogamy, and (5) a tendency to adopt (captive?) children, in order to make family units economically stronger. None of these generalizations are unique to Iban, however. And none seem to be sufficient to explain past Iban expansion.[30]

Afterthoughts

Does good health foster economic development or the other way around? An old view of economists was that improving health increases employment because the population expands as fewer children die and the lifespan increases. The new view is that healthier people are more economically productive. Because healthier people can count on living and working longer, their skills and income will rise over time. In addition, when childhood mortality drops, family size *decreases*, helping to alleviate poverty—a "demographic dividend" provided by better health. To maintain this economic dividend in the face of an AIDS epidemic or the next flu pandemic, however, requires constant investment in health measures.[31]

The game known as rock-paper-scissors in the United States has no single winning strategy. It depends on what one's opponents decide to do. So also in the game of birth-living-death, there is more than one path to well-being or disaster. Fertility and longevity are demographic indicators of well-being but they do not, in the everyday world, equal well-being. Health and laughter are better indicators, far better than a nation's gross domestic product.

In general, human health in Sarawak is changing, largely for the better. The worsening aspects are related to the cash imperative, environmental degradation, and living conditions. These aspects encompass malnutrition, anemia, and some infectious diseases, including sexually transmitted ones. Although not well publicized, the health of Sarawak women is strongly impacted by socioeconomic changes. Children's health, in contrast, has been better monitored and addressed.

---

[30] Because of the tendency to emigrate in kin-structured groups, expansion usually results in a nonrandom genetic makeup of the emigrants, different from that of the original population. This genetic microdifferentiation hypothesis has not been studied in Iban.

[31] Bloom and Canning 2000.

REFERENCES

Abu Bakar Suleiman et al.

1999 A Strategy for Reducing Maternal Mortality. Bulletin of the World Health Organization 77:190–92.

Alexander, J. and P. Alexander

1993 Economic Change and Public Health in a Remote Sarawak Community. Sojourn 8(2):250–74.

2003 Gender and Ethnic Identity among the Lahanans of Sarawak. *In:* Tribal Communities in the Malay World. G. Benjamin and C. Chou, eds. Singapore: Institute of East Asian Studies. Pp. 457–74.

Anderson, A.

1977 Sago and Nutrition in Sarawak. Sarawak Museum Journal 25:71–80.

1981 Nutrition of Iban Children of the Sut and Mujong Rivers. Journal of Tropical Pediatrics 27:26–35.

Andrews, S. and C. M. Wong

2000 Participatory Action Research in a Community Health Development Programme in an Iban Longhouse Community in Sarawak, Malaysia. *In:* Borneo 2000: Environment, Conservation, and Land. M. Leigh, ed. Kuching, Malaysia: UNIMAS. Pp. 385–400.

Annual Statistical Bulletin, Sarawak, 1977

1978 Department of Statistics, Malaysia. Kuching, Sarawak.

Anonymous

1937 Intergovernmental Conference of Far-Eastern Countries on Rural Hygiene. Report of the Preparatory Committee. Geneva: League of Nations Health Organization.

1975 Sarawak Pilot Applied Nutrition Project Baseline Studies Report. Kuching: Department of Medical Services, Department of Agriculture, State Planning Unit, Chief Minister's Office.

1978 Proceeding of the Applied Nutrition Project Seminar/Workshop. Kuching: State Government of Sarawak and UNICEF.

2000a Number of Malaria Cases Up in Sarawak. New Straits Times, June 11.

2000b Africa Must Get Over Sex Taboo to Fight AIDS Scourge. New Straits Times, November 20.

2000c Food Basket Programme Gets RM150,000 Annually. Sunday Tribune of Sarawak, July 2, p. 7.

2001a 4000 Deaths Due to AIDS Since 1986. Borneo Post, July 27, p. 10.

2001b Goal of One Dentist for Every 4,000 by 2020. New Straits Times, September 1, p. 9.

2002 Premarital HIV Testing for Muslims in Malaysia. Population Today 30(1):5.

2004 Highest Number of Breast Cancers Reported in Sarawak. Bernama, April 20.

2005 Remote Penan Tribe Under Quarantine After Measles Kills Fourteen. Malaysiakini, January 24.

Appell, G. N.

1969 Social Anthropological Census for Cognate Societies and Its Application among the Rungus of Northern Borneo. Bijdragen Tot de Taal-, Land- en Volkenkunde 125:80–93.

1980 The Social Separation Syndrome. Survival International Review 5(1):13–15.

1995 Community Resources in Borneo: Failure of the Concept of Common Property and Its Implications for the Conservation of Forest Resources and the Protection of Indigenous Land Rights. Yale Forestry and Environmental Studies Bulletin 98:32–56.

Appleton, A.

2004 Acts of Integration, Expressions of Faith: Madness, Death and Ritual in Melanau Ontology. Ph.D. thesis, Massey University, New Zealand.

Ayob, A. M. and N. F. Yaakub

1991 Development and Change in Batang Ai: Perception of a Resettled Iban Community. Sarawak Museum Journal 42:267–82.

Baer, A.

1998 The Malayo-Borneo Arc: Human Genes vs. Malaria. Borneo Research Bulletin 29:128–42.

1999a Rainforest Malaria, Mosquitoes, and People. Malayan Nature Journal 53(4):299–305.

1999b Health, Disease, and Survival. Subanb Jaya, Malaysia: Center for Orang Asli Concerns.

1999c Indigenous Women's Health. *In:* Asia-Pacific Post-Beijing Implementation Monitor 1999: Health. V. Griffen, ed. Kuala Lumpur, Malaysia: Asia and Pacific Development Center. Pp. 268–78.

2000a Rural Bidayuh and Health. *In:* Borneo 2000: Environment, Conservation and Land. M. Leigh, ed. UNIMAS, Kuching, Malaysia. Pp. 401–16.

2000b Borneo Biomedical Bibliography. Second Edition. Sarawak, Malaysia: Institute of East Asian Studies, UNIMAS.

2001a Rapid Assessment of Rapid Change: Health in Rural Sarawak. Borneo Research Bulletin 32:201–2.

2001b Nutrition. *In:* The Encyclopedia of Iban Studies, V. Sutlive and J. Sutlive, eds. Kuching, Malaysia: Tun Jugah Foundation. Pp. 1291–93.

2003 Health in the Borneo Highlands: The Bario Kelabit. Borneo Research Bulletin 34:87–93.

2004 One Hand Clapping: Malaria in Borneo, Past and Present. Sarawak Museum Journal 81:63–88.

Baer A. et al.

2001 Demography. *In:* The Encyclopedia of Iban Studies. V. Sutlive and J. Sutlive, eds. Kuching, Malaysia: Tun Jugah Foundation. Pp. 444–49.

Barclay, J.

1980 A Stroll Through Borneo. London: Hodder and Stroughton.

Barker, R. et al.

1988 Paediatric Gastroenteritis in the Eastern Malaysia State of Sarawak: An Epidemiological and Clinical Study. Transactions of the Royal Society for Tropical Medicine and Hygiene 82:898–901.

Barnes, G. T.

1966 A Melanau Curing Ceremony (*payun*) at Mukah. Sarawak Museum Journal 14:28–29.

Barrett, R. J.

1993 Performance, Effectiveness and the Iban *Manang*. *In:* The Seen and the Unseen: Shamanism, Mediumship and Possession in Borneo. R. L. Winzeler, ed. Borneo Research Council Monograph Series, Volume 3. Williamsburg, VA: Borneo Research Council. Pp. 235–79.

1997 Cultural Formulation of Psychiatric Diagnosis: *Sakit Gila* in an Iban Longhouse: Chronic Schizophrenia. Culture, Medicine, and Psychiatry 21:365–79.

Barrett, R. J. and R. Lucas

1993 The Skulls are Cold, the House is Hot: Interpreting Depths of Meaning in Iban Therapy. Man 28:573–96.

1994 Hot and Cold in Transformation: Is Iban Medicine Humoral? Social Science and Medicine 38(2):383–93.

Barrett, R. J. et al.

2005 Rates of Treated Schizophrenia and Its Clinical and Cultural Features in a Population Isolate of the Iban of Sarawak: A Tri-diagnostic Approach. Psychological Medicine 35(2):281–93.

Bendell, P. J.
1970 Japanese Encephalitis in Sarawak: Studies on Mosquito Behavior in a Land Dayak Village. Transactions of the Royal Society for Tropical Medicine and Hygiene 64(4):497–502.

Bennett, E. L.
1994 Dance of the Hunters. Wildlife Conservation November/December:56–62.
2000 Timber Certification: Where is the Voice of the Biologist? Conservation Biology 15(2):308–10.

Benster, R. and J. Stanton
1989 Primary Health Care for the Children of Sarawak. British Journal of Hospital Medicine 42:488–90.

Beyrer, C. et al.
1997 Widely Varying HIV Prevalence and Risk Behaviors among the Ethnic Minority Peoples of Northern Thailand. AIDS Care 9(4):427–39.

Bloom, D. and D. Canning
2000 The Health and Wealth of Nations. Science 287:1207–9.

Blust, R.
1995 The Prehistory of the Austronesian-speaking Peoples: A View from Language. Journal of World Prehistory 9(4):453–510.

Bradley, N.
1945 The Old Burma Road. London: Heinemann.

Brooke, M.
1986 My Life in Sarawak. Singapore: Oxford University Press (originally published by Methuen, London, 1913).

Bulan, R.
2003 Boundaries, Territorial Domains, and Kelabit Customary Practices: Discovering the Hidden Landscape. Borneo Research Bulletin 34:18–61.

Burgers, P. et al.
1991 Shifting Cultivation in Teng-Bukap Subdistrict, Kuching Division, Sarawak: A Socioeconomic Study in 16 Communities. Geographical Institute, University of Utrecht.

Burns, A. et al.
1997 Where Women Have No Doctor. Berkeley: Hesperian Foundation.

Calder, R.
1954 Men Against the Jungle. London: Allen & Unwin.

Catterall, R.
1981 Sexually Transmitted Diseases in Sabah and Sarawak. British Journal of Venereal Diseases 57(6):363–66.

Chalmers, L.
1998 Overlaps in the Indigenous Knowledge Traditions of Iban Women. Dialectical Anthropology 23:151–85.

Chandler, G.
1989 Access to Health Care in thc Interior of Sabah. *In:* The Political Economy of Primary Health Care in Southeast Asia. P. Cohen and J. Purcal, eds. Canberra: Australian Development Studies Network. Pp. 101–23.

Chang, M. S. and Nagum Jute
1986 Dengue and Dengue Hemorrhagic Fever Outbreaks in Lawas District, Sarawak, East Malaysia. Medical Journal of Malaysia 41(4):310–19.

Chang, M. S. et al.
1993 Control of Mansonia Mosquitoes, Vectors of Brugian Filariasis in Sarawak, Malaysia. Southeast Asian Journal of Tropical Medicine and Public Health 24(Supplement 2):93–104.
1995 Malaria and Filariasis Transmission in a Village/Forest Setting in Baram District, Sarawak, Malaysia. Journal of Tropical Medicine and Hygiene 98:192–98.
1997 Changes in the Abundance and Behavior of Vector Mosquitoes Induced by Land Use During the Development of an Oil Palm Plantation in Sarawak. Transactions of the Royal Society of Tropical Medicine and Hygiene 91:382–86.

Chen, C. and Raja Latifah R. J.
2000 Knowledge and Perception of Oral Health Promotion in Schools among Dental Nurses in Sarawak, Malaysia. Asia-Pacific Journal of Public Health 12(1):12–16.

Chen, P.
1987 Developing Primary Health Care for a Nomad Tribe: The Penans of Baram. Asia-Pacific Journal of Public Health 1:34–37.
1988a Bringing Leprosy into the Open. World Health Forum 9:323–26.
1988b Longhouse Dwelling, Social Contact, and the Prevalence of Leprosy and Tuberculosis among Native Tribes in Sarawak. Social Science and Medicine 26(10):1073–77.

Chen, S. C.
1985 Agriculture and Resource Utilization in a Lowland Rainforest Kenyah Community. Sarawak Museum Journal 35:1–322.

Chew, D.
1994 Social and Cultural Trends in Sarawak. Sarawak Museum Journal 47:85–100.

Chong Chun Hian
1993 Memoirs of a Pioneer Doctor in Sarawak in the 1950s. Sarawak Gazette 120(1526):5–23.

Chong, G.
1999 HIV/AIDS in Sarawak. Sarawak Gazette 126(1539):12–15.

Christensen, H.
1997 An Ethnobotanical Survey of the Flora Used by Two Longhouse Communities in Sarawak and an Evaluation of their Agronomic Potential for Agroforestry-based Farming Systems. Ph.D. dissertation, University of Aarhus, Denmark.
2000 Economic Importance of Wild Food in a Kelabit Longhouse Community in Sarawak, Malaysia. *In:* Borneo, 2000: Ethnicity, Culture and Society. M. Leigh, ed. Kuching, Malaysia: UNIMAS. Pp. 356–68.
2002 Fallows and Secondary Forests—a Primary Source for Food. Kota Kinabalu: Borneo Research Council.

Chu, G. T. and R. J. Raja Latifah
2001 Utilization of Public and Private Dental Services in Sibu, Sarawak. Asia-Pacific Journal of Public Health 13(2):79–84.

Cohen, J.
2005 Male Circumcision Thwarts HIV Infection. Science 309:860.

Colbourne, M., W. Huehne, and F. La Chance
1989 The Sarawak Anti-Malaria Project. Sarawak Museum Journal 9:215–48.

Colchester, M.
1989 Pirates, Squatters, and Poachers. London: Survival International.

Colwell, R.
1996 Global Climate and Infectious Disease: The Cholera Paradigm. Science 274:2025–31.

Crabtree, S.
1999 Exclusion and Stigma: Implications for Community Psychiatric Services in Sarawak, Malaysia. Asia-Pacific Journal of Social Work 9(1):114–26.
2003 Asylum Blues: Staff Attitudes towards Psychiatric Nursing in Sarawak, East Malaysia. Journal of Psychiatric and Mental Health Nursing 10(6):713–21.
2005 Malaysian Women Service Users and the Economics of the Psychiatric Asylum System. Feminism & Psychology 15(1):87–97.

Crabtree, S. et al.
2001 Community Participatory Approaches to Dengue Prevention in Sarawak, Malaysia. Human Organization 60(3):281–87.

Crain, J. B.
1991 The Anger within the Flesh of the House. *In:* Male and Female in Borneo. V. Sutlive, ed. Williamsburg, Virginia: Borneo Research Council. Pp. 335–44.

Dahaban, Z. et al.
1996 Immediate Effects on Wildlife of Selective Logging in a Hill Dipterocarp Forest in Sarawak: Mammals. *In:* Tropical

Rainforest Research—Current Issues. D. S. Edwards, ed. Kluwer, Netherlands. Pp. 341–46.

Demographic Yearbook, 1992.
1994 New York: United Nations.

Devi, B. C. et al.
2004 High Incidence of Nasopharyngeal Carcinoma in Native People in Sarawak, Borneo Island. Cancer Epidemiology, Biomarkers and Prevention 13(3):482–86.

De Zulueta, J.
1956 Malaria in Sarawak and Brunei. Bulletin of the World Health Organization 15:561–71.
1957 Observations on Filariasis in Sarawak and Brunei. Bulletin of the World Health Organization 16:699–705.

Duffield, A. and S. Strickland
1999 Nutrition in Sarawak: Its Relationship to Rural Development. *In:* Rural Development and Social Science Research. V. King, ed. Phillips, Maine: Borneo Research Council. Pp. 131–58.

Edwards, J.
2000 Reproductive Beliefs and Family Planning Behavior in an Iban Community in Sarawak, Malaysia. MS thesis, University of Alabama.

Elhadi, N. et al.
2004 Prevalence of Potentially Pathogenic Vibro Species in the Seafood Marketed in Malaysia. Journal of Food Protection 67(7):1469–75.

Ellis, D.
1972 A Study of the Punan Busang. Sarawak Museum Journal 20:235–300.

Fauziah Zainal Ehsen and F. Siner Sipeng
1999 The Village Health Promoter Programme in Sarawak. Sarawak Gazette 126(1539):9–11.

Foo, L. C. et al.
1994 Endemic Goiter in the Lemanak and Ai River Villages of Sarawak. Southeast Asian Journal of Tropical Medicine and Public Health 25(3):575–78.
1996 Iodization of Village Water Supply in the Control of Endemic Iodine Deficiency in Rural Sarawak, Malaysia. Biomedical and Environmental Science 9(2–3):236–41.

Friedman, K.
2002 Jungle Fever. Texas Monthly 30(11):244–45.

Geddes, W. R.
1954 The Land Dayaks of Sarawak, a Report on the Social Economic Survey of the Land Dayaks to the Colonial Social Science Research Council. Colonial Research Studies, No. 14. London: Her Majesty's Stationary Office.

1957 Nine Dayak Nights. London: Oxford University Press. Paperback ed., 1961.

George, R. and S. K. Lam
1997 Dengue Virus Infection—the Malaysian Experience. Annals of the Academy of Medicine, Singapore 26(6):8159.

Gerrits, R.
1994 Sustainable Development of a Village Land Use System in Upland Sarawak, Malaysia. Ph.D. thesis, University of Queensland.

Goldblatt, J.
1999 Life after Leprosy. Student British Medical Journal February:28–29.

Gollin, L. X.
1997 Having Your Medicine and Eating it Too: A Preliminary Look at Medicine and Meals in Kayan-Mentarang, Kalimantan, Indonesia. Borneo Research Bulletin 28:28–41.

Gomes, E.
1911 Seventeen Years Among the Sea Dayaks of Borneo. London: Seeley.

Goto, A. et al.
1974 A Survey of Infant Mortality Rates in Sarawak. Southeast Asian Journal of Tropical Medicine and Public Health 5:424–29.

Griffith, G.
1955 Health and Disease in Young Sea Dayak Men. Sarawak Museum Journal 6(5):322–27.

Grijpstra, B. G.
1976 Common Efforts in the Development of Rural Sarawak, Malaysia. Assen, Amsterdam: Van Grocum.

Halliburton, R.
1932 The Flying Carpet. New York: Bobbs-Merrill.

Hang Tuah Merawin
1994 Material Culture in Sarawak: The Sago Connection. Sarawak Museum Journal 47:17–35.

Hardin, S. and A. Kiyu
1991 Child-minding and Nutritional Status of Children 6–12 Months Old in Sarawak. Medical Journal of Malaysia 46(4):338–43.

Harris, A.
2001 Presence, Efficacy, and the Politics in Healing among the Iban of Sarawak. *In:* Healing Power and Modernity: Traditional Medicine, Shamanism, and Science in Asian Societies. L. Conner and G. Samuel, eds. Westport, Connecticut: Bergan & Garvey. Pp. 130–51.

Hatta Solhee and J. Langub
1993 Challenges in Extending Development to the Penan Community of Sarawak. *In:* Restoration of Tropical Ecosystems. H. Lieth and M. Lohmann, eds. Dordrecht: Kluwer. Pp. 239–50.

Heiser, V.
1936 An American Doctor's Odyssey. New York: Norton.

Hew, C. S.
1999 Bidayuh Women and Urban-Rural Migration. Review of Indonesian and Malaysian Affairs 33(1):89–124.

Hew, C. S. and F. Kedit
1987 The Batang Ai Dam Resettlement and Rural Iban Women. *In:* Women Farmers and Rural Change in Asia. N. Heyser, ed. Kuala Lumpur: Asia and Pacific Development Center. Pp. 163–209.

Hew, C. S. and Sharifah Mariam Al-Idrus
1998 Gender Aspects of Labour Allocation and Decision-making in Agricultural Production: A Case Study of the Kelabit in Bario Highlands, Sarawak. *In:* Bario, The Kelabit Highlands of Sarawak. Ghazally Ismail and Laily Bin Din, eds. Petaling Jaya, Malaysia: Pelandok. Pp. 307–30.

Heyser, N.
1992 Rainforest Management and Indigenous Livelihoods: A Malaysian Case Study. Development 4:14–17.
1995 Gender, Population, and Environment in the Context of Deforestation: A Malaysian Case Study. IDS Bulletin 26(1):40–46.

Holden, C.
2005 Sex and the Suffering Brain. Science 308:1574–77.

Horowitz, L.
1998 Integrating Indigenous Resource Management with Wildlife Conservation: A Case Study of Batang Ai National Park, Sarawak. Human Ecology 26(3):371–403.

Hose, C. and W. McDougall
1966 The Pagan Tribes of Borneo. Vol. 2. London: Frank Cass.

Howden, G.
1984 The Cariostatic Effect of Betel Nut Chewing. Papua and New Guinea Medical Journal 27(3–4):123–31.

Hsu, V. P. et al.
2005 Estimate of the Burden of Rotavirus Disease in Malaysia. Journal of Infectious Disease 192(Supplement):S80-S86.

Huang, M.
2002 HIV/AIDS among Fishers: Vulnerability to Their Partners. *In:* Global Symposium on Women in Fisheries. M. J. Williams et al., eds. Penang, Malaysia: ICLARM. Pp. 49–53.

Ireson, C.
1996 Field, Forest, and Family: Women's Work and Power in Laos. Boulder: Westview Press.
Ireson-Dolittle, C. and G. Moreno-Black
2003 The Lao. Boulder, Colorado: Westview Press.
Ismail, M. N. et al.
2002 Obesity in Malaysia. Obesity Reviews 3:203–8.
Jamail, M. et al.
2005 Field Validation of Sensitivity and Specificity of Rapid Test for Detection of Brugia Malayi Infection. Tropical Medicine and International Health 10(1):99–104.
Jensen, E.
1972/73 Sickness and the Iban Manang. Folk 14–15:93–102.
1974 The Iban of Sarawak and Their Religion. London: Oxford University Press.
Jha, P. et al.
2001 Reducing HIV Transmission in Developing Countries. Science 292:224–25.
Joekes, S.
1994 Children as a Resource: Environmental Degradation and Fertility. Focus on Gender 2(2):13–18.
Kamil Mohamed Ariff and Teng Cheong Lieng.
2002 Rural Health Care in Malaysia. Australian Journal of Rural Health 10:99–103.
Kedit, P.
1982 An Ecological Survey of the Penan. Sarawak Museum Journal 30:225–79.
1991 "Meanwhile back home…": Bejalai and their Effects on Iban Men and Women. *In:* Female and Male in Borneo. V. Sutlive, ed. Williamsburg, Virginia: Borneo Research Council. Pp. 295–316.
1993 Iban Bejalai. Kuala Lumpur: Sarawak Literary Society/Ampang Press.
Khor, G. L.
2002 Micronutrient Deficiency and its Alleviation: The Case of Malaysia. Asia-Pacific Journal of Clinical Nutrition (Supplement):S377–S381.
King, V.
1996 Environmental Change in Malaysian Borneo. *In:* Environmental Change in Southeast Asia. M. Parnwell and R. Bryant, eds. London: Routledge. Pp. 165–89.
Kiyu, A.
1985 Epidemiology of Cancer in Sarawak. Southeast Asian Journal of Tropical Medicine and Public Health 16(4):584–90.

1993 Paper No. 9. Bidayuh Cultural Seminar, Volume 2, Session IV. Kuching. Pp. 2–3.

Kiyu, A. and S. Hardin
1992 Functioning and Utilization of Rural Water Supplies in Sarawak, Malaysia. Bulletin of the World Health Organization 70(1):125–28.

Kiyu, A. et al.
1991 Nutritional Status of Children in Rural Sarawak, Malaysia. Southeast Asian Journal of Tropical Medicine and Public Health 22(2):211–16.
1998 Iodine Deficiency Disorders in Sarawak, Malaysia. Asia-Pacific Journal of Clinical Nutrition 7:256–61.

Knapen, H.
1998 Lethal Diseases in the History of Borneo. *In:* Environmental Challenges in South-East Asia. V. King, ed. Richmond, Surrey: Curzon. Pp. 69–94.

Koh, K. H. et al.
2004 A Retrospective Study of Malaria Infections in an Intensive Care Unit of a General Hospital in Malaysia. Singapore Medical Journal 45(1):28–36.

Lam, C. K.
1983 The Population of Sarawak. Ph.D. thesis, Australian National University, Canberra.

Leaman, D. J. et al.
1995 Malaria Remedies of the Kenyah of the Apo Kayan, East Kalimantan, Indonesian Borneo: A Quantitative Assessment of Local Consensus as an Indicator of Biological Efficacy. Journal of Ethnopharmacology 49:1–16.

Lee, D. L. et al.
1999 Intestinal Helminth Infections amongst School Children in the Serian District of Sarawak. Medical Journal of Malaysia 54:96–101.

Leete, R. and K. Kwok
1986 Demographic Changes in East Malaysia and their Relationship with Those of the Peninsula 1960–1980. Population Studies 40:83–100.

Lim, G. C. C.
2002 Overview of Cancer in Malaysia. Japanese Journal of Clinical Oncology 32(Supplement 1):S37–S42.

Lim, T. O. et al.
2000 Distribution of Blood Pressure in a National Sample of Malaysian adults. Medical Journal of Malaysia 55(1):90–107.

Lin Lean Lim
1998 The Economic and Social Bases of Prostitution in Southeast Asia. *In:* The Sex Sector. Lin L. L., ed. Geneva: International Labor Office. Pp. 1–28.

Lin Lean Lim (ed.)
1998 The Sex Sector. Geneva: International Labour Office.

Linklater, A.
1990 Wild People. New York: Atlantic Monthly Press.

Low, W-Y. et al.
2002 Socioeconomic Correlates of Iodine Status among School Children in Sarawak, Malaysia. Asia-Pacific Journal of Public Health 14(2):110–17.

Lye, M. S. et al.
1994 Patterns of Risk Behavior for Patients with Sexually Transmitted Diseases and Surveillance for Human Immunodeficiency Virus in Kuala Lumpur, Malaysia. International Journal of STD and AIDS 5:124–29.

MacKinnon, K.
2005 Parks, People, and Policies: Conflicting Agendas for Forests in South East Asia. *In:* Tropical Rainforests. E. Bermingham et al., eds. Chicago: University of Chicago Press. Pp. 558–82.

Mak, J. W.
1992 Medical Research in Malaysia: Parasitic Diseases. *In:* 90th Anniversary Scientific Seminar: Health Research. Kuala Lumpue: Institute for Medical Research. Pp. 29-69.
1994 Current Malaria Research Activities in Malaysia. Journal of Biosciences (Malaysia) 5:73–79.

Marzhuki, M. et al.
1993 Current Status of Filariasis in Malaysia. Southeast Asian Journal of Tropical Medicine and Public Health 24(Supplement 2):10–14.

Maberly, G. and C. Eastman
1976 Endemic Goiter in Sarawak. Southeast Asian Journal of Tropical Medicine and Public Health 7(3):434–42.

McKay, D. and T. Wade
1970 Nutrition, Environment, and Health in the Iban Longhouse. Southeast Asian Journal of Tropical Medicine and Public Health 1:68–77.

Metcalf, P.
1974 Berawan Adoption Practices: The Tsunami's Psychological Aftermath. Sarawak Museum Journal 22: 275–86.

Miller, G.
2005a Poor Countries, Added Perils for Women. Science 308:1576–77.

2005b The Tsunami's Psychological Aftermath. Science 309:1030–33.

Morris, H. S.
1997 The Oya Melanau: Traditional Ritual and Belief. Sarawak Museum Journal 52:1–388.

Mott, J. A. et al.
2005 Cardiorespiratory Hospitalizations Associated with Smoke Exposure during the 1997 Southeast Asian Forest Fires. International Journal of Hygiene and Environmental Health 208(1–2):75–85.

Nieuwenhuis, A.
1929 Ten Years of Hygiene and Ethnography in Primitive Borneo (1891–1901). *In:* The Effect of Western Influence on Native Civilization in the Malay Archipelago. B. Schrieke, ed. Batavia, Java: G. Kolff. Pp. 10–33.

Nissom, M. P. and K. E. Schmidt
1967 Land Dayak Conceptions of Mental Illness. Medical Journal of Malaysia 21(4):352–57.

Nor Aza Ahmad et al.
1998 Distribution of Intestinal Parasites in a Community of Kelabit School Children. *In:* Bario, the Kelabit Highlands of Sarawak. Ghazally Ismail and Laily bin Din, eds. Petaling Jaya: Pelandok. Pp. 261–66.

Norhanom, A. W. and M. Yadav
1995 Tumor Promoter Activity in Malaysian Euphorbiaceae. British Journal of Cancer 71:776–79.

O'Boyle, S. J. et al.
2002 Factors Affecting Patient Compliance with Anti-tuberculosis Chemotherapy Using the Directly Observed Treatment, Short-course Strategy (DOTS). International Journal of Tuberculosis and Lung Disease 6(4):307–12.

Ogihara, T. et al.
1972a Endemic Goiter in Sarawak, Borneo Island: Prevalence and Pathogenesis. Endocrinology Japan 19(3):285–93.
1972b Serum Thyrotropic Levels of Natives in Sarawak. Journal of Clinical Endocrinology and Metabolism 35(5):711–15.

O'Hanlon, R.
1985 Into the Heart of Borneo. London: Penguin Books.

Oldrey, T.
1972 A Study of the Punan Busang: IV; Medical Report. Sarawak Museum Journal 20:270–77.

Padoch, C.
1982 Migration and Its Alternatives among the Iban of Sarawak. The Hague: Martinus Nijhoff.

Patau Rubis et al.
1981 Parasitological and Entomological Studies on Filariasis in Seven Villages, Serian District, Sarawak. Southeast Asian Journal of Tropical Medicine and Public Health 12(1):30–36.

Pelletier, D.
1992 The Role of Quantitative Methodologies in Nutritional Surveillance. *In:* Rapid Assessment Procedures. N. Schrimshaw and G. Gleason, eds. Boston: INFDC. Pp. 51–59.

Prasad, U. et al.
2002 Long-term Survival of Nasopharyngeal Carcinoma Patients Treated with Adjuvant Chemotherapy Subsequent to Conventional Radical Radiotherapy. International Journal of Radiation Oncology, Biology, and Physics 53(3):648–55.

Quinn, T. and J. Overbaugh.
2005 HIV/AIDS in Women: An Expanding Epidemic. Science 308:1582–83.

Rabi'ah Abdul Ghani and A. Kiyu
1995 Knowledge and Attitudes of AIDS Seminar Participants Regarding Various Aspects of HIV Infection. Sarawak Gazette 122(1533):20–24.

Rashidah Abdullah
1999 Toward Women's Health Needs. *In:* Asia-Pacific Post-Beijing Implementation Monitor: Health. V. Griffith, ed. Asia and Pacific Development Center, Kuala Lumpur, 1999. Pp. 341–45.

Rasit, A. H. et al.
2001 The Pattern of Spinal Tuberculosis in Sarawak General Hospital. Medical Journal of Malaysia 56(2):143–50.

Ridu, R.
1994 Society and Cultural Change: Trends among the Dayaks of Sarawak. Sarawak Museum Journal 47:137–43.

Rintos Mail
2001 Sarawak has Highest Reported STD Cases. The Malaysian Today, 27 June, p. 5.

Rokiah Ismail
1998 HIV/AIDS in Malaysia. AIDS 12(Supplement B):S33–S41.

Sagin, D. D. et al.
2000 Rickettsial Infection in Five Remote Orang Ulu Villages in Upper Rejang River, Sarawak, Malaysia. Southeast Asian Journal of Tropical Medicine and Public Health 31:733–35.
2001 Schistosomiasis Malayensis-like Infection among the Penan and Other Interior Tribes in Upper Rejang River Basin, Sarawak, Malaysia. Southeast Asian Journal of Tropical Medicine and Public Health 32(1):27–32.

2002a Intestinal Parasitic Infections among Five Interior Communities at Upper Rejang River, Sarawak, Malaysia. Southeast Asian Journal of Tropical Medicine and Public Health 33(1):18–22.

2002b Anemia in Remote Interior Communities in Sarawak, Malaysia. Southeast Asian Journal of Tropical Medicine and Public Health 33(2):373–77.

Sarawak Medical and Health Services Department Annual Report

1986 Kuching.

Schmidt, K.

1996 Folk Psychiatry in Sarawak: A Tentative System of Psychiatry of the Iban. *In:* Magic, Faith, and Healing. A. Kiev, ed. London: J. Aronson. Pp. 139–55. (Originally published by Free Press, Glencoe, New York, 1964.)

Schneider, W.

1978 The *biik* Family of the Selako Dayak of Western Borneo. *In:* Sarawak—Linguistics and Development Problems. Studies in Third World Societies Volume 3. Williamsburg, Virginia. Pp. 139–65.

Sellato, B.

1993 Salt in Borneo. *In:* Le sel de la vie en Asie du Sud-Est. P. Le Roux and J. Ivanoff, eds. Thailand: Prince of Songkla University. Pp. 263–84.

Shahar, S. et al.

2001 Social and Health Profile of Rural Elderly Malays. Singapore Medical Journal 42(5):209–13.

Shyamala Nagaraj and Siti Rohani Yahya

1998 Prostitution in Malaysia. *In:* The Sex Sector, Lin L. L., ed. Geneva: International Labour Office. Pp. 67–99.

Simons, R.

1992 Further Skirmishes in the Great Latah Wars. Transcultural Psychiatric Research Review 29:250–55.

Strickland, S.

1986 Long Term Development of Kejaman Subsistence: An Ecological Study. Sarawak Museum Journal 36:117–71.

Strickland, S. and A. Duffield

1997 Anthropometric Status and Resting Metabolic Rate in Users of the Areca Nut and Smokers of Tobacco in Rural Sarawak. Annals of Human Biology 25(3):453–74.

1998 Nutrition and Ecosystem in Sarawak: The Role of the Areca Nut. Asia-Pacific Journal of Clinical Nutrition 7(3/4):300–6.

1999 Biosocial Significance of the Areca Nut in Southeast Asia. *In:* Cultural Food. A. Garcia, ed. Genova, Italy: EGA Edition. Pp. 37–51.

Strickland, S. and S. Ulijaszek
1992 Energy Nutrition of Iban of Song and Kanowit, February-April 1990. Sarawak Museum Journal 43:135–96.
1993 Resting Energy Expenditure and Body Composition in Rural Sarawak Adults. American Journal of Human Biology 5:341–50.
1994 Body Mass Index and Illness in Rural Sarawak. European Journal of Clinical Nutrition 48(Supplement 3):S98–S109.

Sashimi, P. C.
1992 Health and Welfare Services for Elderly People in Malaysia. *In:* Ageing in East and Southeast Asia. D. Phillips, ed. London: Edward Arnold. Pp. 167–84.

Sutlive, V.
1978 The Iban of Sarawak. Prospect Heights, Illinois: Waveland Press.
1991 Keling and Kumang in Town: Differential Effects of Urban Migration on Iban Men and Women. *In:* Female and Male in Borneo. V. Sutlive, ed. Williamsburg, VA: Borneo Research Council. Pp. 489–528.

Sutlive, V. and J. Sutlive (eds.)
2001 The Encyclopedia of Iban Studies. 4 volumes. Kuching: Tun Jugah Foundation.

Talla, Y.
1979 The Kelabit of the Kelabit Highlands, Sarawak. Report No. 9, School of Comparative Social Sciences, Universiti Sains Malaysia, Penang.

Tan Chin Siang
2001 Better Health in Sarawak Now. New Straits Times, 6 August.

Tay, S. T. et al.
2000 Antibodies to Orienta Tsutsugamushi, Rickettsia Typhi and Spotted Fever Group Rickettsiae among Febrile Patients in Malaysia. Transactions of the Royal Society of Tropical Medicine and Hygiene 94:280–84.

Taylor, A. et al.
1986 A Serological Survey of Scrub, Tick, and Endemic Typhus in Sabah. Southeast Asian Journal of Tropical Medicine and Public Health 17(4):613–19.

Taylor, D. et al.
1994 The Degradation of Rainforests in Sarawak, East Malaysia, and its Implications for Future Management Policies. Geoforum 25(3):351–69.

Tee, E. S.
1993 Micronutrient Deficiencies. *In:* Food and Nutrition in Malaysia. E. S. Tee and L. Cavalli-Sforza, eds. Coordinating Committee for the Preparation of the FAO/WHO International

Conference on Nutrition, Rome. Kuala Lumpur: Institute for Medical Research. Pp. 15–45.

Tee, E. S. et al.
1999 School-administered Weekly Iron-folate Supplements Improve Hemoglobin and Ferritin Concentrations in Malaysian Adolescent Girls. American Journal of Clinical Nutrition 69:1249–56.

Then, S.
2003a Dengue Fever Drives Up Demand in Miri Blood Bank. The Star, September 23.
2003b Longhouse Folks Affected by Bakun Project Seek Help. The Star, September 24.

Toynbee, M.
1997 Jungle Schools. Salt Spring Island, British Columbia, Canada: Hepburn.

Voon Boon Hoe et al.
1999 The Nutritional Value of Indigenous Fruits and Vegetables in Sarawak. Asia-Pacific Journal of Clinical Nutrition 8(1):24–31.

Wai, B. H. K. et al.
1996 HIV Infection in Females Dependent on Drugs. Addiction 91(3):435–38.

Walker, J. H.
2002 Power and Prowess. Crows Nest, NSW, Australia: Allen & Unwin.

Wallace, A. R.
1855 Letter. Literary Gazette, June 9, p. 366.
1857 Notes on a Journey up the Sadong River, North-West Borneo. Proceedings of the Royal Geographic Society of London:193–205.
1962 The Malay Archipelago. New York: Dover (originally published by Macmillan, London, 1869.)

Walsh, J. et al.
1993 Deforestation: Effects on Vector-borne Diseases. Parasitology 106:S55–S75.

Wan, K. F. et al.
2003 Antibiotic Resistance, Plasmid Profile and RAPD-PCR Analysis of Entero-pathogenic Escherichia Coli (EPEC) Clinical Isolates. Southeast Asian Journal of Tropical Medicine and Public Health 34(3):620–26.

Wee, C. H. et al.
1996 Poverty, Child Nutrition and Child Care amongst Urban Squatters in Kuching City, Sarawak. Fourth Borneo Research Council Conference, University Brunei Darussalam, June, 1996.

Wells, C.
1925 Six Years in the Malay Jungle. New York: Doubleday.

Wessel, D.
2003 Lessons from Rockefeller's Hookworm War. Wall Street Journal, January 16, p. A2.

Wiebe, P. and A. Rahim Said
1980 Malaysia: Doctors in the Penang General Hospital. *In:* Doctors and Society. T. N. Maden, ed. Sahibabad Dist., Ghaziabad, Uttar Pradesh, India: Vikas Publishing. Pp. 113– 209.

Windle, D. and R. Cramb
1999 Roads, Remoteness, and Rural Development: Social Impacts of Rural Roads in Upland Areas of Sarawak, Malaysia. *In:* Rural Development and Social Science Research: Case Studies from Borneo. V. King, ed. Phillips, Maine: Borneo Research Council. Pp. 215–50.

Winzeler, R.
1995 Latah in Southeast Asia. Cambridge: Cambridge University Press.

Wolffers, I.
1997 Culture, Media, and HIV/AIDS in Asia. Lancet 349:52–54.

Wong, C. M.
1996 Evaluation of a Wakil Kesihatan Kampung Training Course. Kota Samarahan, Sarawak: Institute of Health and Community Studies, UNIMAS.

Wong, C. M. and Abdullah Mohammed
1996 Rural Womens' Reproductive Health Education Needs in Malaysia. Abstract, 23rd Annual Conference Program, National Council for International Health. (Reprinted in Women's Health Weekly 08/05/96, pp. 12–13.)

Wong, J.
2001 Diabetes, Cancer Cases Up. Borneo Post, August 13, p. 1.

Wong, L. M.
1992 Government Dental Services in Sarawak, East Malaysia. Dental Update 19(10):430–34.

Wong, M. L.
1991 Women in Health and Community Development: A Case Study of the Berawans in Sarawak. Singapore: Institute of Southeast Asian Studies.

World Health Organization
1995 Vector Control of Malaria and Other Mosquito-borne Diseases. Geneva: WHO.

WWF (Malaysia)
1985 Proposals for a Conservation Strategy for Sarawak. Report prepared for the Government of Sarawak by the World Wildlife Fund (Malaysia), Kuala Lumpur.

Yaakub, N. F. et al.
1993 Dayak Bidayuh of the Bau-Lundu Region: Demographic profile and Their Perception of Educational Amenities. Sarawak Museum Journal 44:77–91.

Yadav, A.
1994 Low Birth Weight Incidence in Lundu, Sarawak. Medical Journal of Malaysia 49(2):164–68.

Yadav, H. and Chai Meng Chee
1990 Cholera in Sarawak: A Historical Perspective (1873–1989). Medical Journal of Malaysia 45(3):194–201.

Yap, C. P.
1998–1999 Nutritional Assessment of Bidayuh Children Aged 2 to 6 Years in Serian District, Sarawak. B.Sci. thesis, University Putra Malaysia, Serdang.

Yap, S. B.
1985 The Nutritional Status of Iban Preschool Children. Medical Journal of Malaysia 40:185–90.

Yazdanbakhsh, M. et al.
2002 Allergy, Parasites and the Hygiene Hypothesis. Science 296:490–94.

Yearbook of Statistics, Sarawak
2003 Department of Statistics, Malaysia.

Yim, K. S. et al.
1973 Dental Epidemiological Survey of Sarawak School Children. Dental Journal of Malaysia-Singapore 13(1):23–39.

Zain, R. B. et al.
1997 A National Epidemiological Survey of Oral Mucosal Lesions in Malaysia. Community Dentistry and Oral Epidemiology 25(5):377–83.

Zaleha, M. I. et al.
2003 Micronutrients and its Correlation with Mental Performance among Schoolchildren in Bario, Sarawak. Medical Journal Malaysia 58(3):309–19.

INDEX